Working with

with

Adolescent

Voices

John M. Cooksey

SAINT LOUIS

DI017645

Working with Adolescent Voices

TABLE OF CONTENTS

UNDERSTANDING ADOLESCENT VOICES

INTRODUCTION

I. Voice Transformation in Male Adolescents

Voice change in male adolescents presents choral music educators and church musicians with many challenges. It is a complex phenomenon which is not always understood, and there is disagreement among experts regarding the practical applications of current knowledge in the field. Researchers and theorists have studied the process in recent years, and often presented ideas and methodologies quite different in fact and perspective. Prior to the 1970's, prominent experts in the field included Irvin Cooper, Frederick Swanson, and Duncan McKenzie. Dr. Cooper (1965) advocated a Cambiata Plan which took into account the range, tessitura, and shifting tonal quality of the male adolescent changing voice. He further developed his own choral arrangements to suit the unique pitch ranges of the Cambiata voice. Frederick Swanson (1959) proposed that during voice change, most young men's instruments develop first in the lower part of the bass clef, and often have a 'blank spot' between middle C4 and F4 where no notes can be produced. He too developed choral arrangements, demonstrating a much wider pitch range when compared to Cambiata music. The third expert, Duncan McKenzie (1956), presented the Alto-tenor Plan. He viewed voice change as a gradual, sequential process where lower notes appear in the range as top notes gradually disappear. McKenzie's approach allowed for much flexibility in its methodology, and seemed more closely aligned with the views of voice scientists and otolaryngologists of the time.

These experts made significant contributions to the field and helped teachers gain many insights in dealing with adolescent voices. While differing from each other in many respects, there were some points on which they agreed:

1. The voice change occurs at the onset of puberty, and is directly related to the development of primary and secondary sexual characteristics.

2. Most currently published literature is inadequate to fit the range and tessitura of the male changing voice.

3. Irregular growth rates in the vocal mechanism can make the voice unpredictable and difficult to control, particularly if it is forced into the wrong pitch range.

4. In groups of boys between the ages of 12 and 15, one might expect to find voices in many different stages of growth.

5. The rate at which voice changes occur vary with individuals.

6. Individual and group voice testing is necessary.

7. Teachers should help students to understand their voices during the change.

8. It is very important to establish good singing habits during this time.

   The Cooper, Swanson, and McKenzie theories of voice change stimulated discussion and created vigorous debate regarding the description of voice change stages, individual and group voice testing procedures, and recommendations of appropriate choral literature for the changing voice. In answer to these questions, Cooksey (1977 a, b, c; 1978) consolidated findings from empirical and scientific research, and proposed an eclectic but cohesive theory of voice maturation in male adolescents. Utilizing this data, and the Voice Stage Indices of Frank and Sparber (1970 a, b), Naidr, Zboril, and Sevcik (1965), Cooksey, along with speech pathologists, Beckett and Wiseman (1984), designed a longitudinal study to confirm the validity of the **Eclectic Approach.** The purpose of the study was to develop an **Index of Voice Change** and to determine how certain vocal, physiologic, and acoustic factors might define different voice change stages in male adolescents. The results supported many of the previous findings presented by Cooksey in the 1977-78 *Choral Journal* articles and established the validity for his "Contemporary Eclectic Theory of Voice Maturation." Utilizing the criteria of range, tessitura, register development (modal, falsetto, whistle), voice quality (as defined by degree of breathiness and constriction, resonance characteristics), and speaking fundamental frequency (SFF), an Index of Voice Classification was established, and a five-stage process of voice maturation developed. Follow-up studies by Groom (1984), Barresi and Bless (1984), Rutkowski (1984, 1985), Cooksey (1985; 1992–94, 1997, 1998), and Harris, M., Griffin, M., and Hawkins, S. (1996) supported these findings and confirmed the validity of the five stages of voice change in male adolescents.

II. Voice Transformation in Female Adolescents

Voice transformation in female adolescents is a phenomenon which has not held the attention of many researchers over the years; however, there has been relatively significant and increasing interest in the 1980's and 1990's. Researchers and music educators are becoming more aware of the physiological and psychological aspects of female voice change during adolescence. (Alderson, 1979; Brodnitz, 1983; Aronson, 1985; Wolverton, 1985; Fischer and Rose, 1994; Thatcher, 1994; Gackle, 1991, 1997; and Williams, et. al., 1996.) Thurman and Klitzke (1994) report that voice change is one of several signs of female puberty. It appears to begin before menarcheal onset and continues through it. The vocal folds increase in length by about 4mm or 34% (Kahane, 1978), and the vocal tract expands, but not at the rate or dimension of the changing male voice. Most contemporary researchers agree that most girls with changing voices experience the following indicators of voice change:

1. Lowering of the mean speaking fundamental frequency by 3–4 semitones;

2. Increasing breathiness, huskiness, hoarseness;

3. Voice 'cracking' during singing;

4. Noticeable register 'breaks' during singing;

5. Decreased and inconsistent pitch range capabilities;

6. More effort in producing pitches for singing, with a delay in phonation onset;

7. Breathy, 'heavier', 'rougher' voice quality or breathy, thin, 'colorless' voice quality.

To date, there have been no longitudinal studies of the female changing voice, but some comparative research has been done. Cyrier (1981) found that the upper register transition pitch area ('lift point') tends to be higher in 14–15 year old females than in 10–11 year old females. Huff-Gackle (1991; 1997) has also observed this upward trend, identifying specific *passagi* in the voice. In 1987 she examined the effects of selected vocalises on the improvement of tone production in junior high school female voices. By implementing systematic training in breath management, resonation, and vowel unification, the effects of maturation and training could be studied. It was found that, although girls could learn to sing more musically and with greater breath control, breathy tone quality could not be eliminated. During voice change, the folds often do not adduct efficiently enough to achieve full closure.

Finally, Williams et. al., (1996) investigated selected female singing and speaking voice characteristics. The purpose of their study was to compare the speaking fundamental frequency, physioligical vocal range, singing voice quality, and self-perceptions of the speaking and singing voice between two groups of pre- and early adolescent girls, aged 11–15. It was found that symptoms of female vocal maturation generally are manifested in both singing and speaking. Also, both the post-menarcheal and pre-menarcheal groups experienced voice breaks, cracks, pitch changes, inconsistencies in speaking, breathiness, and sore throats from singing. These symptoms increased in post-menarcheal girls.

Huff-Gackle has proposed a three stage pattern of voice development for changing girls' voices: Pre-menarcheal, Post-menarcheal, and young adult phase. While these stages have not been scientifically tested, they should be recognized as a significant step in recognizing and dealing with specific vocal problems of adolescent female singers. These stages, and corresponding implications for voice development will be presented later on in this book. It is important that music educators and all people who work with female changing voices develop

8

more knowledge and awareness of the unique aspects of singing during this time. As a result, these young singers will benefit greatly and be more encouraged to continue their singing activities later on in life.

SECTION 1:

ESTABLISHING A

FOUNDATION

CHAPTER ONE

DESCRIBING THE STAGES OF DEVELOPMENT IN THE CHANGING MALE VOICE

Voice change in adolescent boys is a predictable, sequential, but sometimes erratic process which generally takes place over a period of one to two years. Voices do not change 'overnight,' but develop over time as vocal folds thicken and lengthen, ligament and laryngeal cartilages develop, and vocal tract expansion takes place. The most active phase of change occurs on the average between 12.5 and 14 years of age, but there are many exceptions to this. The most useful criteria for defining the stages of maturation have already been mentioned. These include

- ◆ range
- ◆ tessitura
- ◆ voice quality
- ◆ register development
- ◆ speaking fundamental frequencies

Range is the most reliable of these, but all criteria must be taken into account. Cooksey's Voice Classification System includes the following stages of voice maturation:

Maturational Stage	Voice Classification
—	Unchanged (Pre-mutational)
1	Midvoice I (Early Mutation Period)
2	Midvoice II (High Mutation Period)
3	Midvoice IIA (Climax of Mutation and key transitional period)
4	*New Baritone (Stabilizing Period) *The term "New Voice" is also now being utilized to describe this stage.*

5   *Settling or Developing Baritone
           (Post mutational development and re-
           expansion period)
           *The term "Emerging Adult Voice" is also
           being utilized now to describe this stage.*

*NOTE: The term "Baritone" should not be equated with the adult
          Baritone classification. Young men's voices, while not hav-
          ing adult-like qualities, are nevertheless growing in that
          direction in the Settling Baritone classification. Apparently,
          the young male voice has much developmental potential
          and all evidence points to the fact that growth processes
          continue during high school and college years, and
          beyond.

Figure 1
Mean Ranges and Tessituras for the Voice Change Stages

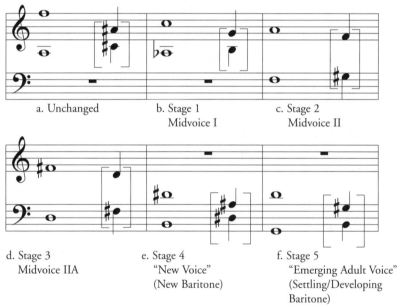

a. Unchanged   b. Stage 1   c. Stage 2
                        Midvoice I   Midvoice II

d. Stage 3   e. Stage 4   f. Stage 5
Midvoice IIA   "New Voice"   "Emerging Adult Voice"
                    (New Baritone)   (Settling/Developing
                                         Baritone)

Bracketed notes—tessituras

Figure 1 shows the mean ranges and tessiturae for the voice change
stages listed above. LTP's (Low Terminal Pitches of the singing range)

show a logical progression downward by thirds. The growth pattern is analogous to a 'slinky' moving down the steps of a stairway! The bottom part of the 'slinky,' or Low Terminal Pitch of the singing range finds the next lower level of the stairway (pitch plateau) and remains stable while the top or High Terminal Pitch (HTP) 'quivers' (becomes unstable) and eventually follows the downward trend. The voice first gains stability in the low to mid-range of each succeeding stage while the upper pitch range generally continues to be unstable. After the voice reaches the fourth stage (New Baritone/New Voice), however, the upper pitch range becomes much more consistent, and by the fifth stage (Developing Baritone/Emerging Adult Voice) the growth process has slowed down considerably. Here, there is more stability generally in the voice as the range begins to expand.

The growth pattern described above is highly correlated with the development of primary and secondary sexual characteristics associated with puberty. The onset of voice change, Stage 1,–Midvoice I, begins as the physiological changes take place. Higher pitches are lost (usually between C5–F5) and the singing range decreases by about four semitones. While high notes may still be produced for a while, there is increased constriction and breathiness. There is also an overall decrease in the richness of the tone. The first stage begins between the ages of 12 and 13, but can occur sooner (11 to 12 years of age), and may last for several months or continue for more than a year. Individual growth rates vary, so one can not predict how long adolescent singers will remain in this stage.

In the Stage 2–Midvoice II, following the 'slinky' effect, lower pitches begin to appear in the adolescent's range while higher notes become much more unstable. Primary and secondary sexual characteristics are more evident. This signals the beginning of the second maturational stage of voice development, Midvoice II. As the lower pitch plateau is established at the E3/F3 level below middle C, HTP's (A4-C5) begin to fluctuate and the falsetto register begins to emerge. Register lift points appear, and because of transition adjustments between the two registers, some coordination can be lost. On the other hand, some voices have no trouble with this and can even produce notes in a whistle register. Figure 2 shows typical ranges for the modal, falsetto and whistle registers.

Figure 2
Typical Ranges of Registers: Midvoice II

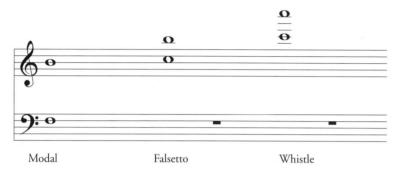

Modal   Falsetto   Whistle

Voice quality in the Midvoice II classification is distinctive—thicker, darker in color, and less resonant. The most stable pitch area is between A3 and F4.

For most adolescents, this stage lasts for about 12–13 months, and begins closer to 13 years of age. Again, there are many exceptions. Some boys may remain in Midvoice II for a few months, while others for several years.

Voice change reaches a high point in Stage 3–Midvoice IIA. This is the time when the voice is most vulnerable to abuse. Few vocal parts published in standard choral literature fit the range of this unique stage. LTP's descend to D3 (below middle C), and average HTP's occur at about F4. The falsetto register continues above this point, but in some cases is not easily produced, particularly in the area just above the highest pitch in the modal range. The most comfortable part of the singing range is limited to G3–C4/D4. The quality of the voice is huskier than Midvoice II, and has a tendency towards breathiness. There is also a loss of agility, and boys want to 'push' or force the tone sometimes, especially in the lower and upper pitch extremes. Midvoice IIA is a transition stage and may last for only 4 weeks, or in some cases between 2 and 10 months. (There are, of course, exceptions to this.) The majority of Midvoice IIA's are found in the eighth grade. The normal age span of boys in this classification is 13–14 years of age.

15

The Stage 4–New Baritone/New Voice period represents the beginning of more stability in the voice change process, for the most dramatic period of maturation is over. While the range is stable (B♭2/B2-C4/D4), the voice quality is clearer but remains light and somewhat thin. The sound does not approximate adult-like quality. The New Baritone/New Voice has less pitch agility, but usually produces the falsetto register fairly easily. In some cases, however, there is a 'blank spot' (C4–F4) where no notes can be produced at all. Some may experience difficulty in 'finding the falsetto.' Others can sing falsetto very easily above F4, but cannot produce pitches below that point without pushing or forcing tone in the modal register. Register transition vocalises may help, but sometimes it is best to be patient and not 'force' the issue. In most cases this situation will improve as the voice gains further maturity. In the Cooksey, et.al. Study, this stage lasted an average of 3–5 months, but in some cases varied between 4 weeks and 8 months. A large percentage of New Baritone/New Voices can be found in both the eighth and ninth grades. Normal mean age for this classification is 14 years of age, but can vary between 13–15 years of age.

The Stage 5–Developing Baritone/Emerging Adult Voice classification, represents a marked tendency towards vocal maturity. Adult-like characteristics are still not apparent, but unique voice qualities begin to appear. There is a gradual expansion in range and vocal capability, and more consistency in vocal production generally. The falsetto register is very clear and 'focused,' while the register transition area, D4/E4, is slightly lower than New Baritone/New Voice. Developing Baritone/Emerging Adult Voices can sing most bass parts, but their optimum pitch area is B♭2–A3. At this stage of maturation, there is dense growth of pubic and auxilliary hair in body development. Chest and shoulder dimensions continue to increase, as does weight, height, and vital capacity. Vocal folds have reached maximum length, and vocal tract cavities are approaching completed size and configuration. Regarding the speaking voice, SFF's appear in some cases 4–6 semitones above the LTP of the vocal range. In voice change stages, fundamental frequencies averaged about 2–4 semitones above the LTP's of the vocal range. All in all, these voices are more flexible and generally easier to work with in the choral setting. The Developing Baritone/Emerging Adult Voice is prominent among ninth grade boys, and begins at approximately 14–15 years of age.

NOTE: For further information and a more complete summary of each of the voice change stages, consult Appendix A.

In summary, voice change is a predictable phenomenon which follows a rather logical sequence of events. The various stages can be defined in terms of specific criteria: range, tessitura, register development, voice quality, and speaking voice fundamental frequency. Throughout the period, from early, middle, climax, tapering, to postmutational stage, range parameters are generally consistent, but HTP's vary more than LTP's. The overall width of the range contracts about four semitones initially, and does not expand again until the Developing Baritone/Emerging Adult Voice Stage. Vocal tessituras move towards the middle and lower pitch areas of the singing voice range, but may vary considerably from individual to individual. The falsetto register becomes evident during Midvoice II but is sometimes difficult to produce. Distinct voice qualities emerge for each of the voice change stages, but there is an overall loss of vocal richness and fullness. Amplitude of spectral partials is much weaker when compared to the premutational stage. Changing voices become less agile, and more vulnerable to vocal abuse. Finally, the speaking voice pitch (SFF) averages about 2–3 semitones above the Lowest Terminal Pitch of the singing voice range, then gradually goes to 4–6 semitones above LTP by the postmutational period.

How does the church youth choir deal with multiple stages at one time? There are many ways to insure success. Helpful methods have been developed for auditioning singers, classifying voices, assigning singers to parts, setting up seating arrangements, developing good tone production, applying vocalises in the rehearsal situation, and selecting appropriate music for changing voices. After a brief discussion of girls' changing voices, practical applications in these areas will be presented.

CHAPTER TWO

DESCRIBING THE STAGES OF DEVELOPMENT IN THE CHANGING FEMALE VOICE

Mirroring aspects of adolescent male changing voice research, Huff-Gackle (Gackle, 1987) has proposed developmental stages for the female changing voice:

Stage I:	Prepubertal (Unchanged)
Stage IIA:	Pre-menarcheal
Stage IIB:	Post-menarcheal
Stage III:	Young Adult Female

Even though her system does not parallel the nomenclature utilized by Cooksey with changing male voices, it is helpful to realize that the focal points of change come basically within three stages or periods, Pre-menarcheal, Post-menarcheal, and Young Adult Female. While these stages have not been tested longitudinally, they are grounded in extensive experience and research-in-action. They provide a starting point for further study and may well become the foundation structure for a tested theory on female adolescent voice development. Huff-Gackle (1997) uses the following criteria in classifying female voices:

◆ average speaking voice pitch

◆ total vocal range and range of tessitura

◆ register 'breaks' (quality changes)

◆ voice quality

These are the same criteria which Cooksey utilized in determining the various changing male voice stages; however, it is very clear that the criteria of voice quality, register breaks, and tessitura range are very important in describing female stages. This is because the range of the female singing voice does not fluctuate significantly as voice develop-

18

ment proceeds. This obviously presents more challenges to choral conductors, for they must be more sensitive to subtle aspects of change in
female singers. Figure 3 shows ranges and tessiturae for each stage,
while Figure 4 shows lift point areas, indicating register transitions or
shifts in the natural vocal mechanism.

Figure 3
Mean Ranges and Tessituras for the Female Voice Change Stages

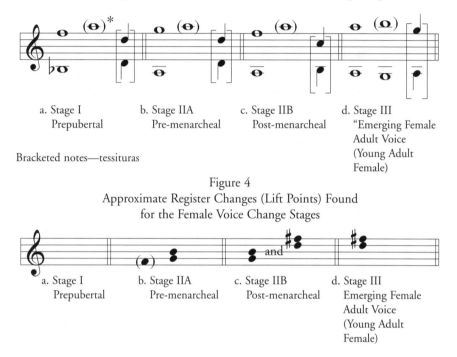

a. Stage I	b. Stage IIA	c. Stage IIB	d. Stage III
Prepubertal	Pre-menarcheal	Post-menarcheal	"Emerging Female Adult Voice (Young Adult Female)

Bracketed notes—tessituras

Figure 4
Approximate Register Changes (Lift Points) Found
for the Female Voice Change Stages

a. Stage I	b. Stage IIA	c. Stage IIB	d. Stage III
Prepubertal	Pre-menarcheal	Post-menarcheal	Emerging Female Adult Voice (Young Adult Female)

In the Stage I–Prepubertal, the female voice is much like its counter-
part, unchanged male, but is often perceived as lighter in 'weight'
because the volume potential is generally not as great (Gackle, 1997:
p. 585). There are no apparent register breaks, and the voice has a
light, flute-like quality. It is flexible and able to handle intervallic
skips. This stage is evident during 8–10/11 years of age, and, depending upon physical maturation and menarchy, could continue to 11 or
12. When listening to these voices, one must be careful to disallow
oversinging in any parts of the range. Sometimes belting, for example,
will produce an illusion of register change from lower parts of the
range to upper pitch areas.

Stage IIA–Pre-menarcheal (pubescence), may begin between 11–12/13 years of age. This is the beginning of mutation when the first signs of puberty and physical maturation occur. As mentioned earlier, breathiness increases noticeably and singing can become difficult and at times uncomfortable. There is difficulty in achieving loudness (especially in the middle and upper range) and, while a fuller tone can be achieved in the lower range, obvious changes to the breathy, child-like tone occur at transition points from lower to upper registers. The lower/upper register break appears between G4 and B4 (around a fifth above middle C) and, if not utilizing the lower voice very much, there is an apparent loss of lower range notes around C4 (middle C). Some girls have trouble producing the lower register at this time. While breathiness is obvious, the quality of the voice is fuller than those 'child-like' tones of unchanged voices; however, the tone qualities are generally 'thin' (lacking in full resonance) among singers going through this initial or early stage of development.

Stage IIB–Post-menarcheal (puberty), begins between the ages of 13–14/15 at the peak of mutation (Ruble, 1982). After Stage IIA, tessiturae can move up or down, or sometimes can narrow, yielding basically a five or six note range of 'comfortable singing' (Gackle, 1992: p. 410). Register breaks are still common in several key areas (Fig. 4, page 15). Gackle states that,

> At times, lower notes are more easily produced, yielding an illusion of an 'alto' quality; singing in this lower range may be easier and can be recommended for short periods of time; (however) singing only in the lower range for an indefinite period can be injurious to the young 'unsettled' voice because of a tendency to overuse the lower register. Vocalization throughout the singing range will help vocal development, avoiding any unnecessary strain in the lower or upper range. (1992: 410-412).

Williams et. al. (1996) reports that girls in this stage have a better understanding or awareness of the effects of voice development. They report that they experience less control, particularly in the speaking voice. The researchers found that these inconsistencies occurred more often during this stage and that the general symptoms of voice change were more evident. As with boys' changing voices, some girls experience these problems in a more pronounced way, while others seem to move through the stages with relative ease.

Stage III–Young Adult Female (Emerging Female Adult Voice), usually begins somewhere between the ages 14–15/16 and signals the end to much of the instability of the female changing voice. Overall range capabilities increase and breathiness decreases. There is now more consistency between registers. The tone is richer and occurs with greater ease. Vibrato may appear and there is an increase in volume and vocal agility. Another facet of adolescent female voice change is reported by Williams et. al. who found that their post-menarcheal sample (11–15 years) had lower speaking voices than their pre-menarcheal subjects.

In summary, the female voice follows a somewhat predictable but uneven path in voice development during adolescence. While ranges do not change noticeably, register shifts occur in transition areas which can be very unstable. As the female laryngeal apparatus grows, vocal fold coordinations become more difficult, and comfort zones in the singing voice can appear in diverse pitch regions. As with males, the onset and length of time within stages is highly variable. Individual growth rates vary considerably. Vocal quality often becomes breathy (see also Williams et. al., 1996 who also reported incomplete closure of the posterior vocal folds in their post-menarcheal subjects) and individuals may experience various forms of constriction, especially in the midrange area. Female voices are highly vulnerable during the height of change and should be cultivated carefully during this time.

SECTION 2:

APPLICATIONS

IN THE

YOUTH CHOIR SETTING

CHAPTER THREE

ASSIGNING VOICES TO PARTS: GROUP AND INDIVIDUAL CLASSIFICATION PROCEDURES

Figures 1 (p. 13) and 3 (p. 19) show that the church choir director may have a youth choir filled with boys and girls in many stages of vocal growth. This is particularly true if there are a number of 7th and 8th graders in the ensemble. Due to time constraints, the director can apply a Group Voice Classification procedure that will allow singers to be assigned to their proper parts at the very first rehearsal. This technique is NOT a substitute for hearing each person individually! Voice classification should be done on a person-by-person basis as time permits.

If there are young people in the choir who are older, and know their voice classification, it would be wise for them to observe the group procedure. They can easily be included in the latter stages of the part assignment process.

GROUP VOICE CLASSIFICATION

1. Divide the class into two groups, with boys together in one section, and girls in the other.

2. Ask everyone to sing "America" ("My Country 'tis of Thee") in the key of C. The keys of B or B♭ will also work, particularly if there are a number of 'more mature' boys in the choir. The range of a 6th fits the vocal ranges reasonably well for all parts. Another 'limited range' song may be used, but if so, be sure that it does not extend below B♭3 (just below middle C4), nor above G4 or A4. The girls and the Midvoice I's and II's sing in the *treble clef compass* with some of the II's overlapping into the bass clef. New and Developing Baritones (New Voice, Emerging Adult Voice) will sing the melody one

octave lower than the other voices. Midvoice IIA's may sing more easily in the upper part of their ranges.

3. Ask the boys to sing "America" as a group in the key of C (or B♭/B). Listen for voices singing in the octave BELOW C4. As you walk around, touch the shoulders of the boys who are singing in the lower octave, and afterward, ask them to stand together and sing the song through again. Listen again. Some Midvoice IIA's will sing pitches just above C3, and therefore may be assigned to a baritone part. Some IIA's, however, may still sing in the upper octave. Assign these to the tenor part (if the choir is SATB). Also, listen for boys singing in the falsetto register during this process. Some Midvoice II's and even New Baritones/New Voices may do this. When in doubt, check their ranges!

   In cases where boys are not matching pitches, listen for notes sounding below the target pitches. Boys who 'err' below the target pitches may be developing the ability to be pitch accurate with their growing voice. Boys who are not yet really baritones will 'sound' above the target pitches that are being sung by the majority.

4. Seat the baritones as a section in their own area.

5. Ask the remaining boys to sing "America" in the key of F or G. Walk through the section and tap the shoulders of the boys who are obviously singing in the upper octave *with ease*. Also note the lightness of the vocal quality. These should be Midvoice I's and Unchanged voices. Ideally, Unchanged voices will be more successful vocally if they sing the soprano part, and Midvoice I's should be assigned to the alto part in a mixed SATB chorus. Midvoice I's can be assigned to a tenor part that does not go below G3 or A3. Ask these boys to stand as a group and sing "America" again, listening for boys who are actually further into the change process, but are singing in falsetto register. These boys may be baritones or Midvoice II's!

Boys are very self-conscious in the 7th and 8th grades, and in a mixed choir situation, they do not want to be identified with any 'high' or 'soprano' part. Careful psychological preparation, choice of terms, and straightforward explanations of the change process may help them 'reframe' the 'negative' connotations. In a male choir, the group dynamics change, and there is more flexibility in assigning these voices to 'higher' parts.

6. The remaining voices should be Midvoice II's and IIA's. Ask them to sing "America" in the key of B♭, with their beginning note as B♭3 (just below middle C). If necessary, let them sing once more to 'solidify' their accurate pitch singing, then ask them to take their seats together as a section. In an SATB choir, they would be assigned to the tenor part. Careful selection of music for this part is crucial. If the line goes below E3 or F3, the part will be too low.

7. For the girls, ask them to sing "America" in C or B♭. Touch the shoulder of the girls with the 'strongest,' most 'clear' voices, who are producing their tones with relative ease. Then have all the girls sing the song in the key of F or G, and again touch the shoulders of the girls who are singing clearly, strongly, and with relative ease but not 'forcing.'

8. Singers who were touched in both keys, may be divided evenly into two sections. Voices that sing with relative ease in only the upper or only the lower keys may be assigned accordingly. The remaining girls with 'weaker' voices may be assigned evenly between the two sections. Note that girls' voices are also changing at this age, and are not at all like adult soprano or alto voices.

9. Ask the two groups of girls, one after the other, to sing "America" in both keys, B♭ and G, and then together in the two keys. Listen for uniformity of tonal quality and balance within and between the groups. There should not be a great difference in quality or volume between the two sections.

In summary, the primary criteria for part assignment with girls are:

1. clarity and strength of sound in both upper and lower ranges;

2. location of vocal tessiturae; and

3. voice quality.

   Accordingly, girls in Sections I and II may either (or alternately) sing soprano and alto parts, providing ranges in those parts are not extreme.

10. Finally, everyone sings "America" in C (B♭, B) to establish a feeling of unity and confidence. High school singers may join in at this point.

11. When using a group classification procedure in an all-boys group, the changing voice classifications can be telescoped into three subgroups:

   A.) High (Unchanged and Midvoice I)
   B.) Middle (Midvoice II and Midvoice IIA)
   C.) Low (New Baritone/New Voice and Developing Baritone/Emerging Adult Voice)

Seating Arrangements for Changing Voices

After completing the group classification procedure, the director can consider a number of ways for seating the singers. Chart A shows how changing voices can be organized in a mixed choir situation.

CHART A

Girls 1	All Baritones	Midvoice IIA	Midvoice II	Unchanged Midvoice I Girls 2

The above seating arrangement enables the director to have easy access to all sections of the choir. The conductor can move into the group to help singers with their parts, to listen to boys in each section, and always be ready to move voices as they change. Overall composition of the voice parts will change as the year progresses, with more and more boys progressing through the various stages. Unchanged and Midvoice I's will be few in number by Spring!

Chart A can also be adapted to choirs, grades 7-12. Consider the following placement:

CHART B

Senior High School Sopranos Junior High School Girls 1 Some Unchanged Boys	Senior High School Basses Junior High School New/Settling Baritones	Senior High School Tenor I,II Junior High School Midvoice II, IIA	Senior High School Altos Junior High School Girls 2 Midvoice I Some Unchanged Boys

Chart B shows that it is relatively easy to group junior and senior high singers so that individual needs can be met. Notice that the junior highs are placed in front of the high school singers. This insures less 'pushing' or 'forcing' from the younger singers.

28

Chart C shows yet another way to group junior and senior high school voices.

CHART C

Senior High School Sopranos	Senior High School Altos	Senior High School Tenors	Senior High School Basses
Junior High School Girls 1 Unchanged Boys	Junior High School Girls 2 Midvoice I	Junior High School Midvoice II, IIA	Junior High School New/Settling Baritones

This arrangement is also very flexible, and changing male voices can be moved easily in order to sing parts with appropriate ranges. With the men grouped together, confidence will grow, but care must be taken to preserve a healthy balance with the lighter women's voices. Charts A and B are a little more effective in this regard.

It is not always wise to 'mix' (intersperse) junior high singers with senior high singers in seated and standing arrangements (such as mixed quartet formations). Junior high singers will try to compete with the more mature singers, and this can cause vocal problems to develop which will affect the tone quality of the choir as a whole. In any case, ALL singers should be encouraged to sing without forcing the tone. Junior high singers should be valued for their own unique capabilities and should not be encouraged to sound more mature than they really are. If the director will apply sound principles of healthy tone production, changing voices will develop in the most beneficial way.

INDIVIDUAL VOICE CLASSIFICATION

It is not unusual for the LTP (Low Terminal Pitch) of the male singing voice range to drop 1–2 semitones every three to four weeks. However, rates among individuals vary considerably. With such rapid voice development individual testing should be done at least every 6–8 weeks. It is therefore advisable for the youth choir director to create a Range Chart for each male adolescent singer. In this way, both the director and young person can keep track of vocal changes as the year progresses.

In the individual audition, other factors besides range should be assessed. Some of these include tessitura, voice quality (degree of breathiness, constriction, resonance), register development (when and where falsetto begins), Speaking Fundamental Frequency (SFF), posture and breath control, volume capabilities, dynamic-rhythmic agility, pitch agility, tonal memory, diction, intonation, outstanding personality characteristics, and vocal strengths and/or weaknesses. While the list is long, these criteria can be tested in a very short period of time. The Individual Audition Form in Appendix C shows how some of this information can be organized. To evaluate the junior high male singers using the criteria listed, the youth choir director may consider the following procedures:

1. **Student enters room.** The student should have completed the general information section of his audition card. (This provides the director with information about the singer's musical background: choral and instrumental experience, private study, etc...) Talk to the young person to put him at ease. Call him by name and ask him questions about his interests in and outside of school (athletics, hobbies, etc...) By carefully listening to the quality and pitch level of his speaking voice, the director can get some idea of where to begin matching tones. After experience is gained in listening to the speaking voices of boys in the various stages, characteristic qualities and pitches can be identified more readily. To find a good starting pitch from the speaking voice, ask the young man to count backwards from twenty. He should recite the numbers slowly and at a steady rate. The average speaking voice pitch (SFF) will be about 2–4 semitones above the LTP of the singing voice range. Starting pitches may be given in the general area of the SFF. The following starting pitches and SFF's are commonly found in each of the voice change stages for the male adolescent voice:

Stage	Average SFF's	Best Starting Pitches for Singing
Unchanged	A3/B3	C4–A4
Midvoice I	A3/B♭ 3	C4–G4
Midvoice II	A ♭3	B♭3–C4
Midvoice IIA	F♯3	G3–B♭3
New Baritone/New Voice	D3	D3–G3
Developing Baritone/ Emerging Adult Voice	B♭2/B2	B2–F3

NOTE: It is a decided advantage to begin singing in a pitch range where the singer has a chance for immediate success. Boys at this age need much encouragement and positive reinforcement.

2. **Matching pitches.** Ask the young man to stand a few feet from the piano facing you but unable to see the keyboard. Boys should keep their eyes on the director so that they will not 'psych' themselves out as the notes go higher. After finding the best starting pitch area, ask the singer to sing an open vowel 'AH' on a sustained note. Encourage him to project the sound with energy and confidence. Watch for the tight jaw and the failure to open the mouth properly.

3. **Determine voice classification and range.** If the young man matches initial pitches, begin to move in stepwise fashion down, then up the scale, testing for Low Terminal Pitches (LTP) and High Terminal Pitches (HTP) in the range. Be sure that the singer sings an open vowel and smoothly connects the notes. (Open vowels are utilized to reveal more of the full resonance of the voice and identify register changes.) Do not insert consonants from pitch to pitch. Listen carefully for register changes in the upper part of the range. Also check for undue tension in the neck area.

The director can expect the Midvoice I to show some strain in the C5–F5 area. Because the falsetto register becomes clearly recognizable in the Midvoice II stage, listen for the change in quality particularly in the G4–C5 pitch area. For Midvoice IIA, register lift points will occur often in the D4–A4 range. For New Baritone/New Voice, lift points occur often between D4 and F4, and Developing Baritone/Emerging Adult Voice has lift points between C4 and G4. The important thing is to listen carefully for the regular normal sound, rather than changes in quality for the falsetto range. This is a key element in healthy voice placement and management. Finally, make note of the range and register change pitch areas, and determine the correct voice classification for the singer.

4. **Tessitura, etc...** To check for tessitura, diction, vocal problems, breath control, volume, and intonation, ask the young man to sing "America" in the proper pitch range. The following keys are suggested:

Unchanged:	E4, F4, G4
Midvoice I:	D4, E4
Midvoice II:	B♭3, B3, C4 (possibly)
Midvoice IIA:	G3, A♭3, F3 (possibly)
New Baritone/New Voice:	C3, D3, E3
Developing Baritone/ Emerging Adult Voice:	B♭2, B2, C3

5. **Flexibility exercises.** Now try some quick flexibility exercises. Sing the 1–3–5–3–1 exercise on 'pah' ascending and descending by half steps using the same sequence. Again, be careful to stay within the pitch ranges suggested by the Cooksey Classification System. (see p. 13)

6. **Tonal memory test.** Play three-note, stepwise patterns and ask singers to sing them back to you. Then go for triads and gradually work for larger intervallic separations.

7. **Rhythmic memory, sense of tempo.** Use a call/response technique, clapping simple quarter, half, and eighth note patterns. The singer listens and claps the patterns in tempo and sequence, not losing the feeling for the basic pulse. Next, use dotted patterns, rests, then syncopations. Go to two measure sequences, using the same method.

All of these results can be recorded easily on an audition form, but more importantly, valid, reliable individual voice assessments insure the possibility for future successful singing and vocal development.

For junior high girls the same steps and basic procedures should be followed; however, there are some differences. The following chart lists the SFF's and appropriate starting pitches for girls: (Gackle, 1991)

Stage	Average SFF's	Best Starting Pitches for Singing
Prepubertal	C4/D4	C4–E4
Pre-menarcheal	B5/C♯4	C4–D4
Post-Menarcheal	A5/C♯4	C4–D4
Young Adult Female	G♯5/B5	B5–E4

In general, as one listens to each individual, significant attention should be placed on the criteria of tessitura, voice quality, and register shifts. The Unchanged voice has a fairly wide tessitura (See Figure 3), sounds very light and a little breathy, and, unless overcompressing (belting), has no apparent register shifts. The Pre-menarcheal voice maintains a fairly wide tessitura, has a significant increase in breathiness, and displays a discernable shift in registers between G4 and B4. Some individuals may have trouble singing notes in the lower pitch range. The Post-menarcheal voice has register changes between G4 and B4, and between D5 and F♯5. The tessitura is variable and can move

33

up or down, or narrow at either end of the range. Sometimes the lower range sounds fuller giving the illusion of an 'alto' sound. The quality of the tone will vary, depending upon the register. Cracking and breathiness frequently occur. Much of the instability of voice change is gone as the Young Adult Female voice emerges. The tone will be clearer, fuller, and the tessitura will be wider. Some vibrato may appear, and there is more consistency between registers. Overall, it may be more difficult to hear subtle differences between these stages than with changing male voices. It is important, however, to exercise these female voices throughout their ranges so that consistency can be cultivated with the tone production. In light of this information, care should be exercised to allow girls to experience singing both alto and soprano parts. If girls are placed strictly on the alto part, they will not have the opportunity to develop their full range, or attain healthy tone production.

CHAPTER FOUR

UNISON SINGING

After voices have been classified and sections established, the choir is ready for vocalises and part singing. Because of the complexities of working with voices in perhaps 5 to 6 different voice classifications, the youth choir director should become aware of some of the problems of unison singing. In general, because most tunes cover over an octave in pitch range, it is not possible for changing male voices to sing all the pitches. Major compromises therefore have to be made, range-wise, for this activity. First of all, try to find songs with a limited range of a major sixth. Then choose a key which will fit the recommended composite range for Unchanged, Midvoice I, II, IIA, New Baritone (New Voice), and Developing Baritone (Emerging Adult Voice). Figure 5 shows the Composite Unison Range for Unchanged and Changing Voices.

Figure 5
Composite Unison Range
for Unchanged and Changing Voices

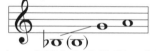

Unchanged, Midvoice I, II, IIA and Girls

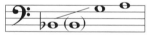

New and Developing Baritones

It is still difficult in certain ways for some changing voices to sing in the Composite Unison Range. Notes around F4–G4 are high for Midvoice II. Midvoice IIA may want to drop an octave in the upper pitch areas, and Unchanged voices may find the Composite Unison Range somewhat low.

The director should also note that vocalises should begin in the Composite Unison Range, but can be expanded upward, depending on the skills developed by changing voices in utilizing the falsetto register.

Unison singing (including vocalises sung by all sections at the unison octave) *can* benefit the choir. If proper caution is taken in selecting limited range tunes, if each singer knows his/her own range limitations and sings 'intelligently' without forcing, unison singing can be utilized to:

    a. aid in pitch-matching exercises;
    b. aid in developing proper tone/energy/breath support for singing;
    c. aid in teaching concepts of phrasing and dynamics;
    d. aid in the conductor quickly establishing rapport, 'conducting' technical control of a new choir; and
    e. aid in teaching concepts of expressive singing, including elements of control and refinement in the tone.

Limited range songs are difficult to find, especially those which begin close to middle C. The following tunes have been utilized effectively with changing voices:

Song Title	Key Structure
"America"	C, B, or B♭
"Sweet Afton"	E♭, E
"Deck the Halls"	C
"Coventry Carol"	Cm
"When the Saints Go Marching In"	B♭ or B
"Oh, Come, Oh, Come, Emmanuel"	Em
"Rocky Mountain High"	B or B♭
"I Hardly Think I Will"	B or B♭
"Captain Jinx"	E
"San Sereni" (Portugese folk song)	B♭
"Kum Ba Yah"	B or B♭
"Our Boys Will Shine"	E♭ or E
"Ain't My Susie Sweet"	B or B♭
"For He's a Jolly Good Fellow"	B or B♭

CHAPTER FIVE

EXERCISING THE VOICE IN ITS MATURATIONAL STAGES

Principles to Consider

1. *Establish good habits of proper posture and breathing for singing.*
   Because of the continuing growth of the chest cavity, the larynx
   and pharynx, and associated muscles during puberty, proper coordination for phonation is sometimes difficult to achieve. It is vitally
   important to teach adolescent males proper concepts in this area.

2. *Utilize kinesthetic movement as an essential element of warmups and
   choral singing.* The body's physical, emotional, and intellectual
   response are released through appropriate movement activities.
   Adolescent singers need to become more aware of how the 'felt'
   experience of physical responses to music affects vocal performance
   and the enjoyment of singing activities.

3. *The proper coordination between the sub-glottic air pressure, extrinsic
   and intrinsic muscular control of the vocal folds, and articulation
   within the resonance areas must be achieved.* It is important to secure
   the correct balance between air pressure, vocal fold resistance, and
   overall energy level input into the sound as the voice passes
   through its various stages of maturation. If too much air pressure is
   applied, the folds can not approximate properly and excessive tension is created within the laryngeal muscles to compensate. This
   happens often during the most active phases of change: Midvoice
   II, IIA. Excessive air flow will only tend to increase the mild hyper-
   tension associated with vocal fold approximation during the climax
   of voice change.

4. *Begin vocal exercises in the most comfortable singing area of the range.*
   Expand the range after proper concepts of tone production are
   achieved.

5. *As the voice develops, be sure that enough vocal practice is given in the
   proper modal register.*

6. *Educate adolescent singers about the physiology and acoustics of singing and speaking.* Teach them to understand the process of voice maturation. Teach them about the signs of stress and tension in singing. Inform students about their own vocal capabilities.

7. *Teach adolescent singers to LISTEN!* They can tell when forcing the tone occurs. They should be able to hear good pitch and know when flatting and sharping occurs.

8. *Range extension and handling of the falsetto register can be accomplished.* Care must be taken to establish proper principles of good tone production. The development of the transition area between modal and falsetto register can be especially troublesome for changing voices.

9. *Do some separate exercises for the female voice which encourage tone development throughout the range.* Arpeggios and top/down vocalises are excellent ways to accomplish this development.

10. *Proper exercises can be developed to improve pitch agility.*

11. *Work for precise vowel and consonant articulation.* Be sure that young singers do not 'overdo' articulatory movements.

12. *The director should begin working with the comfortable singing range and tessitura which each individual has, regardless of the variety of stages in the youth choir situation.* It is important to consolidate the comfortable middle range through each voice stage so that hyper-functional habits can be avoided. This does not mean that the voice should only sing in one area. Care should be taken, but singers may perform in the lower and upperparts of their ranges. To accomplish this, work on a section by section basis, at least part of the time in each choral rehearsal. Cultivate the light mechanism in transition areas between the modal and falsetto registers, and choose music which will fit the ranges of changing voices.

13. *Always look for visible and audible signs of vocal stress.* Devise techniques for dealing with these problems.

14. *Don't practice for long periods of time.* This will cause vocal stress and fatigue.

15. *Be sure to 'spotlight' the changing voice in a positive manner.* It is a healthy, natural phenomenon. Young adolescents will be very 'accepting' of these changes if the director is confident of his/her knowledge of voice maturation.

Teaching Good Posture and Breathing

One of the most important and vital parts of voice development is the breath management process. Healthy singing takes place with good body alignment and coordinated use of air pressure with laryngeal function. If voices are exercised properly utilizing efficient breathing techniques, beautiful, resonant tone can be achieved. To build a foundation for good tone and healthy singing, the folowing techniques for teaching good posture and breathing are recommended.

Posture

With proper posture it is possible to insure increased efficiency of the vocal and breathing mechanism.

> For good posture, the head, chest, and pelvis should be supported by the spine in such a way that they align themselves one under the other, head erect and chest high. The position of the head and shoulders allow the jaw to be free, not pulled back into the throat. This liberates the organs in the neck. The high chest implies that the shoulders go back, but they should be relaxed and comfortable. (Cooksey, "Changing Voices," Choral Journal., 1977, Dec., p. 12).

To teach the above concepts:

1. Ask everyone to stand, spacing themselves apart at arms length from each other.

2. Rest the body weight easily on slightly parted feet. Watch out for feet which are too close together, or aligned exactly evenly. One foot should be placed slightly in front of the other.

3. Raise the body and stretch the arms from the sides to an elevated position at right angles to the body. This should be

done slowly until the arms are even to the shoulder level. Simultaneously and slowly elevate the body on tip-toes.

4. Slowly return to normal position, keeping the arms outstretched. The arms should lower as the body goes to its original position. During this process, keep the chest elevated and shoulders back. The weight of the body should rest evenly on both feet in the original standing position. Be sure the body does not tense or become 'locked' in a soldier-like, stiff position.

5. Rotate shoulders now, relax the body, but maintain high chest position and upright body stance. With good body alignment (erect head, high chest, shoulders back, arms at sides, and balanced body position), the young adolescent is ready to sing with maximum efficiency.

Breath Management

Because of the continuing growth in the size of the thorax and associated muscles (intercostal, diaphragmatic, and abdominal) during puberty, proper coordination between these muscles during singing is difficult to achieve.

The act of breathing involves at least two major phases, inspiration and expiration (inhalation and exhalation). During inspiration, the thorax expands, and the lungs fill with air from the bottom lobe to the top. As air fills the lungs, the walls of the thorax (chest) expand, aided by the upward pulling of the external set of intercostal muscles. The slope of the ribs is such that pulling them up moves the sternum forward and also expands the rib cage sideward. Simultaneously, the diaphragm (large dome shaped muscle that provides a floor for the thorax and separates the heart and lungs from the abdominal viscera) contracts and lowers itself, increasing the capacity of the thorax. When the diaphragm drops, it presses down upon the stomach viscera, thus encouraging muscular abdominal expansion. In the expiratory phase, the internal intercostal muscles pull the ribs of the chest back into place; the abdominal muscles (four sets), resisted and steadied in their contraction by the diaphragm, compress the viscera, causing it to press against all the abdominal surfaces (including the diaphragm). If the fibers of the diaphragm are relaxed, the visceral pressure will push the diaphragm upward to decrease the thoracic

40

area, increase the internal pressure, and thus force the air out. (1977, Dec.,p. 11)

To teach this concept to the youth choir, it is suggested that a clear, concise explanation of proper breathing be given. One might draw a figure (see Figure 6), or present a video on how the chest expands, the stomach relaxes and expands, and the diaphragm lowers/contracts during inhalation, and how the intercostal muscles aid in this process.

Figure 6

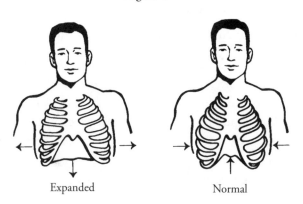

Expanded   Normal

Upon exhalation, show how the thorax returns to normal position. Make the point that one can not feel the diaphragm, and that there is a slight squeezing action felt just below the sternum (epigastrium muscle area) continuing down to the lower abdominal area as exhalation occurs.

The following breath management exercise begins from deep breathing and progresses logically to normal breathing for singing. Be careful that students remain relaxed in the upper shoulders and neck area during the exercise, and that they do not 'try too hard,' to take in too much air during inhalation.

1. Place the palm of the hand on the area of the stomach just below the sternum (epigastrium area) or upper abdominal region. This allows adolescents to physically monitor the expansion and contraction muscular process that occurs during inhalation and exhalation.

NOTE: During the following steps, the conductor should show through his/her gesture when to breathe and for how long. That is, move the arms apart to indicate inhalation and then bring them back together during exhalation (outward from body, then back). Be sure to make the entire action continuous and do not stop action between inhalation (full air capacity reached) and exhalation. Young people, at the end of exhalation, have a tendency to lock the muscles in the neck and stomach region if they 'hold' the air back just before letting it out again.

2. Exhale air first by hissing, 'sssss' (or use the 'ffff' consonant).

3. Upon release of abdominals after exhalation, inhale by audibly sucking air in through puckered lips. (This controls the rate of air flow going into the lungs, and permits the chest and abdominal area to expand gradually.) Guard against excessive throat tension here. Inhale slowly and evenly. You may wish to count to four, or show how long you want inhalation to last by indicating this with your conducting gesture.

   At the end of inhalation, immediately expel the air by hissing, 'sssss.' (Do not lock the throat area or tense abdominal muscles unduly at the moment just before expiration; also, do not hold or lock the air just before exhalation.) The entire inspiration and expiration process should be thought of as a continuous action.

4. Repeat...checking for relaxation in the upper part of the body, particularly in the throat and stomach regions during inhalation.

5. Suck the air in (on a reverse 'hiss')...then connect with a voiced (sung) sound, 'sah.' The hiss, upon exhalation, may take place for a count or two, after which the 'sah' sound begins, or one may choose to phonate immediately. The 'sah' tone should be a comfortable note for all voices. If a mixed choir is participating in this exercise, use middle C (octave below for baritones). If you are working with individuals or sections, use F4 for Unchanged voices, Midvoice I's; middle C or B♭3 for Midvoice II's, IIA's, F3 or E3 for New and Developing Baritones.

6. Inhale (sucking the air in); expel the air on whispered 'hah.' This eliminates the lip area as the focal point for expelling the air, and allows the singer to feel the upward flow of air in the back of the throat area.

7. Inhale on whispered 'ah' and expel on whispered 'hah.'

8. Inhale on a whispered 'ah,' and connect immediately upon expiration with the sung sound, 'hah,' on a comfortable tone. (See Figure 5 p. 35)

9. Gradually eliminate the whispered 'ah' (inhalation) so that a normal, noiseless inspiration of air is accomplished. Along with the elimination of inspiratory air noise, there should develop a well-coordinated intercostal, diaphragmatic-abdominal action which serves to direct the air pressure at the proper rate and intensity through the glottis. The resulting tone should be rich and unforced.

10. Try steps 7–9 at different tempos.

11. As a separate exercise, do the above sequence slowly, on a whispered 'ah,' 'hah.' Gradually speed up until the singer is panting on one breath...then integrate additional staccato exercises.

It may take several sessions, particularly in a large ensemble to go through all the steps outlined above. Not everyone will catch on right away, so individual help sessions will be necessary. Key problems regarding breathing will appear with some individuals.

1. *Failure to hold the chest up; relaxing the abdominal area during inhalation.* Solution: Reinforce good posture (e.g. Stretch and raise arms high above the head and gradually lower them maintaining a relaxed upper body position.) Place hand on middle or lower stomach area and gradually inhale through the mouth feeling the expansion of the stomach as the lungs fill with air. Do not 'try too hard.' Also, concentrate on expelling the air first (on the 'fff' consonant sound), releasing the abominal muscles as inhalation simultaneously occurs.

43

2. *Shallow breathing: too much chest action; raising shoulders.* To solve this problem, move the shoulders during inhalation and relax. Another technique: in the sitting position stretch the body by pulling elbows forward over the knees. Inhale slowly, feeling the expansion in the lower back area. In a standing position, lean over, with arms and head relaxed (floppy), and slowly inhale and exhale. Return to standing position, and inhale/exhale feeling lower back expansion. (Hands may be placed in back to feel this action.) Finally, try touching the top of the shoulders with hands (arms in curved positon) while breathing. This makes the singer aware of excess movement, and minimizes muscular tension in the shoulder and chest region.

3. *Reverse muscular action; stomach pulls inward as singer breathes.* To solve this problem, place the student's hand on your upper stomach (just below the sternum), and your hand on his; then breathe together. If the singer is sensitive to being touched, ask him to place his own hand on yours (which is placed on your own stomach), and your hand on his hand (which is located on his own abdomen). As you breathe together, he will quickly catch on that the stomach must *relax* to expand outwardly during inhalation. One might also apply some pressure inward upon the student's abdomen during exhalation so that the 'release' of the stomach muscles (sudden outward expansion) for inhalation are felt more precisely. Another solution: Move arms outward from the body during inhalation, with the stomach following the arm movement (imagery). (Beginning position: holding an imaginary baby.) As the singer exhales, the arms follow the stomach back (moving inward towards the body, back to the original position.

With proper emphasis and follow-through, techniques of good posture and breathing will produce healthy singing in young adolescent singers. The youth choir will improve its tone production, and individuals will learn more about their vocal capabilities, and develop a thorough understanding of the basics of singing. It is very important to place a strong emphasis on posture and breathing, for these are the areas which *must* be under control if changing voices are to develop in the healthiest manner possible.

KINESTHETICS AND VOCAL WARMUPS

There are a number of vocal and physical exercises which are beneficial in preparing adolescents for vocal singing. These activities are important because movement is an essential part of the body's reaction to music. Alperson (1974) identifies two levels of response to music. The first level is a 'felt' experience. That is, the body experiences or feels the process of making music. "This level relates to the right hemisphere of the brain which controls spatial awareness, artistry, body cognizance, and recognition of faces." (Dickson, 1972, p. 17). The second level, the symbolic level, relates to the left hemisphere of the brain, "involving analytical thinking, language, and logic." (Dickson) This allows the adolescent to conceptualize, analyze, and develop perceptual awareness of the 'felt' experience; therefore, kinesthetic (movement) activity in vocal warmups can be extremely beneficial in encouraging efficient and creative bodymind responses to music.

Emphasis might first be placed upon physical activities during warmups. Through this activity adolescents can become more aware of body conditioning as a preparation for vocal activity. Thus the whole body is energized for singing, and mental alertness and focus are achieved. It therefore becomes easier to sing more efficiently and to be able to transfer some types of movement and physical energy to vocalises and choral singing.

SOME SUGGESTED PHYSICAL ACTIVITIES

A. Stretching Exercises

(Always check for possible tension in neck, shoulders, stomach, arms, legs, etc...)

1. Reach up, slowly, one arm first, then the other, and stretch. Do both arms, and stand on the balls of your feet, balancing the entire body. Gradually allow the arms to come down at right angles to the body while simultaneously bringing the heel down to a normal position. (See Section on Posture p. 39)

2. Inhale, exhale, with arms up, then down. Check head/neck relationship and muscle involvement in the shoulders, back and abdomen regions.

3. Place left arm over the area above the elbow of the right arm, and gently stretch or pull using the left arm. Turn the body towards the left as you do this. Reverse arms, and pull the right arm and body in the opposite direction.

4. Lift right arm then left arm vertically and stretch as if picking fruit from a tree. Make the motions continuous with several repetitions.

B. Body Relaxation Activities

1. Shake the left hand vigorously, feeling the effects on the tip of the fingers. Do the same for the right hand, then both together. Shake the left leg, and if brave, shake the left leg and both arms! This is lots of fun and will bring some laughter.

2. Neck: locate joint where the head rests on the spine. Roll head, checking the amount of neck movement. Change the alignment of the body to the motion of the head in the neck area.

3. Close eyes and do some slow, deep breathing.

4. Do some hand patting exercises beginning on the lower leg and coming across the abdomen and going down the other leg. This encourages the entire body to relax.

5. Do some light jogging in place. Keep the body relaxed. This will stimulate the entire body and prepare it for vigorous singing activities.

C. Bending

1. Bend forward and check where you bend—from the hip or the back. Make sure the head 'hangs' and is not locked in place. Gradually return to normal position.

2. Bend forward and inhale, exhale several times in this position. Check involvement of abdominal muscles, back muscles, rib cage, etc... Now rise slowly and compare the breathing sensation in the upright position to the sensation in the bend position.

D. Brain/Body Coordination

1. 'Shake' arms/legs and change combinations.

2. Walk in place, with left hand touching the right knee; right hand touching the left knee in sequence to a moderate beat.

3. Do a variety of hand jives, and other motions such as clapping and gesturing which require the participants to do these exercises simultaneously with you and in delayed sequence.

E. Facial Warmups

1. Massage temple, cheeks, jaw, neck, tongue base, etc...

2. Make faces: East/West vs. North/South for example. Be creative: Invite the singers to make their faces look like prunes, or as wide as the globe. Ask for happy, sad, angry faces, etc... Elicite responses from them. This can really be a 'fun' activity.

TRANSFERRING MOVEMENT SKILLS TO VOCALISES

Vocalises can be presented for building good tone quality and resonance, building intervallic agility/dynamic control, rhythmic flexibility, managing smooth register transitions, and extending range. Movement which is incorported in these exercises can enhance creative and efficient body responses to music. The feeling of motion in time and space can be translated into a vocabulary of physical responses to music. (Dickson, p. 18). Adolescent singers therefore utilize gesture and full body movement to focus on the 1) design, 2) direction, and 3) density (Dickson, Ibid) of the musical score or vocalise. Dickson relates design to the visual graphing of the musical phrase followed by

47

gestures silhouetting the shape or contour of the line. Through self-guided movement and choreography students gain greater insight into the spatial dimensions of music. (Dickson, Ibid). In discovering and feeling 'direction' in music, students can differentiate through movement the vertical and horizontal aspects of music. Physical movements primarily involving hand and upper body gestures can reflect linear and vertical patterns and convey more rhythmic styles. Finally, *density* conveys the sense of weight between beats—a 'pulling' motion which involves varying degrees of intensity. For example, the gesture might include the right hand and left hand moving on a horizontal plane in opposite directions reflecting the degree of intensity in the musical phrase.

Movements can be very effective not only in expressing aspects of singing but also in enabling young singers to increase vocal efficiency and encourage healthy body alignment and breathing. Smooth arm movements on a horizontal plane can encourage a relaxation response. Vertical staccato beat gestures can enhace evenness in octave leaps as long as the body alignment remains consistent. For vertical, rhythmic patterns, small staccato beats (gestures) encourage less weight in the sound. Arm motions going in opposite directions from ascending and descending pitches encourage throat relaxation and consistent tone quality. This is particularly effective in arpeggios and scalar patterns. Knee bends can produce more upper body and throat muscular release if executed for the top notes of arpeggios. It is apparent that the creative use of gesture and body movement enhances tone production by eliminating unnecessary points of tension and stress in the body. It is up to the teacher and students to develop their own ongoing vocabulary of movements to enhance good tonal production. This prevents the 'locking' or tightening of muscles and stiffness of body frequently seen in young singers.

Suggestions will be made in the Vocalise Section of this book for movement options, but these are only a few ideas. Teachers and students are encouraged to develop their own movements which seem appropriate for each vocalise.

VOCALISES FOR THE CHANGING VOICE

Once the principles of good posture, breathing, and kinesthetic activity have been established, vocalises can be utilized much more effectively. As vocalises are applied, the following principles should be considered:

1. *All vocalises should be carefully explained and applied.*

2. *Utilize the Composite Unison range at first, beginning on B♭3/B3/C4, performing sustained vowels on one pitch, then moving gradually to ascending/descending four note scalar patterns.*

3. *Mix staccato/agility exercises with more sustained exercises in each rehearsal.* This will allow voices to develop tremendous pitch flexibility in a very short period of time.

4. *Emphasis should be placed on full body involvement, kinesthetics, and the basics of good posture and breathing.* Emphasize above all, freedom and relaxation in the upper chest, head, throat, neck, and chin areas. Encourage appropriate physical movement as an essential part of singing. Be creative in exploring body movements appropriate for each exercise.

5. *Find the 'optimum' sound for the full choir and each section. The tone should be energetic, projected, and vibrant, without being 'pushed' or 'forced.'*

6. *Utilize exercises which 'release' the voice, and encourage 'mf,' 'f' levels of dynamics at first.* This is much easier with young changing voices; do not go for 'control' at the 'pp' level immediately.

7. *Be consistent and spend adequate time each day with these exercises.*

8. *Be creative and devise new vocalises each day.* Don't always repeat the same ones.

The vocalises presented in the following section should be applied with the whole choir and on a section by section basis. This will insure the full vocal development of each individual, regardless of voice change stage. The director should therefore mix group and sectional work during the warm-up period. Figure 7 shows the recommended separate (sectional) composite ranges and tessituras for each section of the choir. Refer to Figure 5 p. 35 for the Composite Unison Range for all voices.

Figure 7
Composite Ranges, Tessiturae for Each Section of the Youth Choir Grades 7–12*

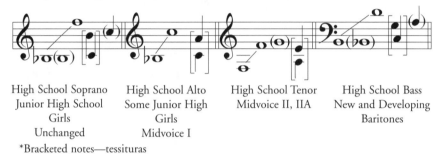

High School Soprano	High School Alto	High School Tenor	High School Bass
Junior High School Girls	Some Junior High Girls	Midvoice II, IIA	New and Developing Baritones
Unchanged	Midvoice I		

*Bracketed notes—tessituras

Vocalises will now be presented in the following areas:

Building Good Tone Quality and Resonance
Sustained fundamental vowels
Energizing tone
Improving vowel consistency and resonance
Balance in articulation between air pressure and vocal fold function

Building Intervallic/Dynamic, Rhythmic Flexibility
Precise articulation and pitch agility
Dynamic control
Rhythmic flexibility

Register Transitions and Range Extension
Modal to falsetto and vice versa
Passagio (Register transition) control

BUILDING GOOD TONE QUALITY AND RESONANCE*

Sustained, Fundamental Vowels

1.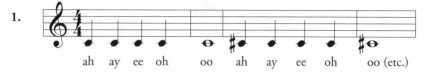

ah   ay   ee   oh   oo   ah   ay   ee   oh   oo (etc.)

Continue each sequence up by half steps to E4 or F4, then descend by half steps to C4 or B3.

2.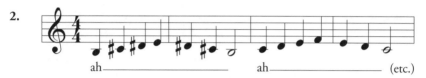

ah——————————— ah——————————— (etc.)

Repeat above sequence utilizing other fundamental vowels: Ay, ee, oh, oo. Also utilize combinations of vowels. Continue to ascend by half steps until top pitch of A4 is reached, then descend by half steps to original starting point. (NOTE: 'Top pitch' in above context means the HIGHEST pitch reached within each sequence or tonal pattern.)

Movement Activities:

1. Use horizontal hand/arm motions moving to the left and right, adhering to the beat/tempo of the music.

2. Try circular, smooth hand motions going with the beat/tempo of the music.

3. Sway the body gently, left and right, to the beat/tempo of the music

*These exercises should also be implemented on a section-by-section basis utilizing appropriate ranges/tessiturae for each part. (see Figure 7 p. 50).

All New and Developing baritones should sing these vocalises one octave lower.

Energizing Tone

1.

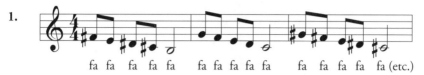

fa fa fa fa fa   fa fa fa fa fa   fa fa fa fa fa (etc.)

Also try syllables 'bah' and 'vah.' Continue each sequence up by half steps to top pitch of about A4, then descend by half steps to starting pitch, B3.

2.

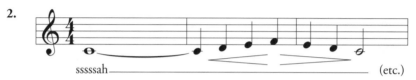

sssssah ———————————————————————————————— (etc.)

Continue each sequence up by half steps to top pitch of A4, then descend by half steps to starting pitch, B3.

3.

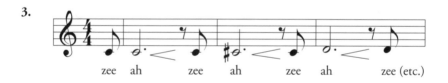

zee ah   zee ah   zee ah   zee (etc.)

Continue each sequence up by half steps to F4, then descend by half steps to B3.

4.

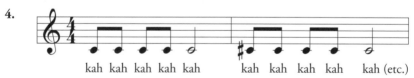

kah kah kah kah kah   kah kah kah kah   kah (etc.)

Continue each sequence up by half steps to top pitch of F4, then descend by half steps to B3. Utilize comfortable tessiturae when individual sections sing this exercise. Encourage accenting 'k.' Sing exercise with 1–2–3–4–3–2–1 pattern (♩=60). Repeat sequence up by half steps to top pitch of G4, then descend by half steps to original starting point, or lower to B3, B♭3.

5.

yah yah yah yah   yah   yah yah yah yah yah (etc.)

Continue sequence up by half steps to G4, then descend by half steps to original starting point, or lower to B3, B♭3.

Movement Activities:

1. For exercise one, flick fingers out, very lightly to the beat; conduct small quarter note patterns; gesture each quarter note with an appropriate hand motion.

2. For exercise two, utilize a pulling, horizontal motion with a closed hand, suddenly releasing or opening the hand when the vowel is sounded.

3. For exercise three, apply the same motions as suggested in two. Choose variations on this.

4. For exercise four, conduct light, staccato patterns. Utilize strong energy with the hand motion but maintain a small pattern.

5. Utilize circular patterns with the right arm; make smooth patterns according to the phrase sequence.

Improving Vowel Consistency and Resonance

1.

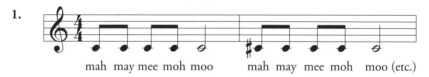

mah may mee moh moo   mah may mee moh moo (etc.)

Continue sequence up by half steps to F3, then descend by half steps to B3, B♭3.

Sing the exercise above utilizing other pitch sequences: e.g. 1–2–1–2–1,1–2–1–2–1, (up by half steps, descend by half steps, etc...) or 1–2–3–2–1, 1–2–3–2–1, (up by half steps, descend by half steps, etc...).

2.

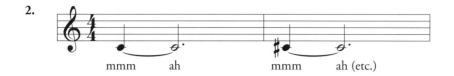

mmm ah mmm ah (etc.)

Continue sequence up by half steps to F4, then descend to B♭ 3. Keep soft palate high and throat open when the 'ah' vowel is sounded. Utilize other fundamental vowels: 'mmm ee,' 'mmm ay,' 'mmm oh,' 'mmm oo.' Also utilize 1–2–3–4–3–2–1 tonal pattern with 'mmm ah,' etc... vowels.

Ex.

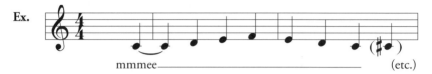

mmmee (etc.)

Up by half steps, down by half steps, (etc...)

3.

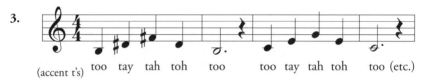

(accent t's) too tay tah toh too too tay tah toh too (etc.)

Continue sequence down by half steps to starting pitch of B♭3. Stress position of articulators (lips, and tongue especially); try additional patterns.

4.

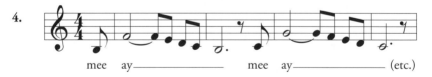

mee ay———— mee ay———— (etc.)

Continue sequence, descend by half steps to starting pitch of B♭3 or A3. Try other combinations of vowels: 'mee ah,' 'mee oh,' 'mee oo.'

5.

lug-ged- dy lug- ged- dy lug-ged- dy lug- ged- dy   lah (etc.)

Continue sequence up by half steps, then descend by half steps to
B♭3. This exercise is good for resonance, low larynx, flexible jaw, and
the tongue. This helps get rid of excessive nasality.

Movement Activities:

1. For exercise one, apply smooth horizontal gestures.

2. For exercise two, apply single direction, sustained hand/arm
   movements. Keep the energy and intensity at a high level.

3. For exercise three, conduct light, staccato beats.

4. For exercise four, apply downward, half circular gestures.
   Make these rather large and smooth. Keep the feeling of continuous movement in the gesture.

5. For exercise five, do a standard four-beat conducting gesture.

Balance in Articulation between Air Pressure and Vocal Fold Function

1. Staccato

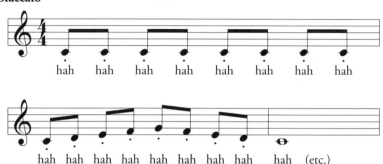

hah hah hah hah hah hah hah hah

hah hah hah hah hah hah hah hah   hah (etc.)

Continue sequence, down by half steps to beginning pitch of B♭3. Do this lightly. Place hand on epigastrium area to feel the bounce of the stomach. As sections do this exercise, utilize their most comfortable ranges. Try above exercise using 1–1–1–1–1–1–1–1 1–3–5–3–1 pattern.

2.

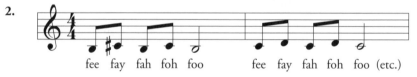

fee fay fah foh foo   fee fay fah foh foo (etc.)

Continue sequence by half steps up to the top pitch of F4, then descend by half steps to starting pitch of B♭3. Emphasize the consonant 'ffff' sound.

3.

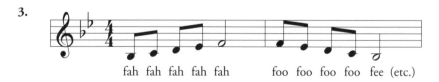

fah fah fah fah fah   foo foo foo foo fee (etc.)

Continue sequence up by half steps to the top pitch of G4, then descend by half steps to starting pitch of B♭3. Try other combinations of vowels and stepwise patterns.

Movement Activities:

1. For exercises one and two, conduct light, short vertical gestures, on the beat.

2. Conduct a light, small beat pattern on the quarter notes but sustain and lift the hand from the ictus on each half note.

BUILDING INTERVALLIC/DYNAMIC/RHYTHMIC FLEXIBILITY

Precise Articulation and Pitch Agility

1.

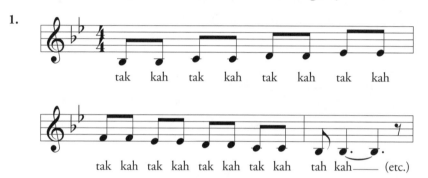

Try this sequence with the beginning pitches of B3, C4. This exercise is good for precise articulation, pitch agility, and energy. Try above exercise with the following pitch pattern:
1–1–3–3–2–2–4–4–3–3–2–2–1.

2.

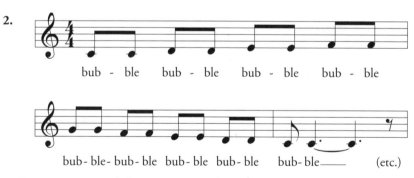

Sing exercise with beginning pitches B♭3, B3.

3.

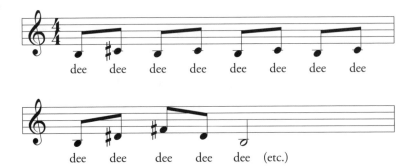

dee   dee   dee   dee   dee   dee   dee   dee

dee   dee   dee   dee   dee   (etc.)

Continue sequence up by half steps to top pitch of G4, then descend by half steps to starting pitch of B♭3.

4. Staccato

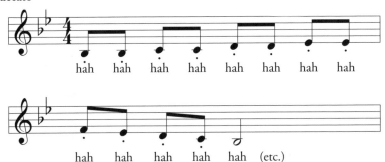

hah   hah   hah   hah   hah   hah   hah   hah

hah   hah   hah   hah   hah   (etc.)

Sing exercise with beginning pitches B3, C4.

Movement Activities:

1. Emphasize vertical gestures, short downward thrusts, on the beat; light vertical hand movements.

Dynamic Control

1.

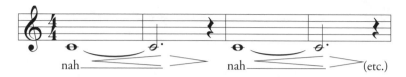

nah⎯⎯⎯   nah⎯⎯⎯   (etc.)

Continue sequence up by half steps to F4; then descend by half steps to B3. Try other syllables: 'noh,' 'noo,' 'nee,' 'nay.'

2.

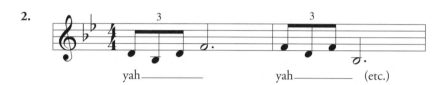

yah⎯⎯⎯⎯   yah⎯⎯⎯   (etc.)

Repeat sequence in keys of B, C. Try other syllables: 'yoh,' 'yoo,' 'yee,' 'yay.'

3.

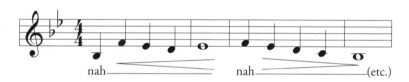

nah⎯⎯⎯⎯⎯   nah⎯⎯⎯⎯   (etc.)

Repeat sequence in keys of B, C. Try other syllables: 'noh,' 'noo,' 'nee,' 'nay.'

Movement Activities:

1. Continous, smooth right and left hand movements on a horizontal plane; size of the gesture should parallel the dynamic levels indicated in the exercise.

2. For exercise two, apply half and full circular movements of the hand.

3. For exercise three, apply smooth, horizontal conducting patterns per half note.

Rhythmic Flexibility

1.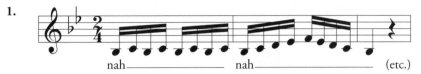

nah———————— nah———————— (etc.)

Continue sequence up by half steps until top pitch of G4 is reached, then descend by half steps to starting point of B♭3.

Movement Activities:

1. Apply light, staccato gestures on quarter note beats.

REGISTER TRANSITIONS AND RANGE EXTENSION: UTILIZING MODAL AND FALSETTO REGISTERS

NOTE: Caution should be taken so that throat, jaw, and upper body tension is held at a minimum in these vocalises. Some changing voices can produce pitches in certain areas of the falsetto register. Others have difficulty in producing tones, particularly between C4 and G4. Individuals should relax as much as possible. These 'problem' areas will disappear generally after the main activity of voice change is completed.

1. Falsetto to Modal Transition

a. For Midvoice II, IIA

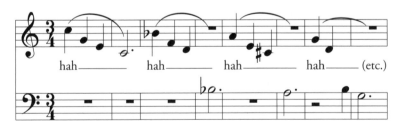

hah——— hah——— hah——— hah——— (etc.)

Yawn-sigh exercise, top down. Begin on aspirated 'H'

b. For New and Developing Baritones (New Voices; Emerging Adult Voices)

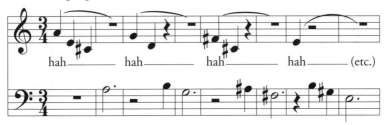

hah_____ hah____ hah____ hah_____ (etc.)

Substitue 'noo' (closed vowel) in the exercise above. This is a very effective way to make smooth transitions between registers.

2. Falsetto to Modal, back to Falsetto Transition

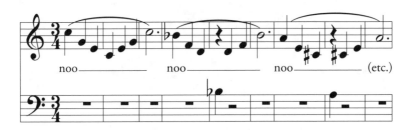

noo_____ noo_____ noo_____ (etc.)

a. For Midvoice II, IIA

b. For New and Developing Baritones (New Voices; Emerging Adult Voices)

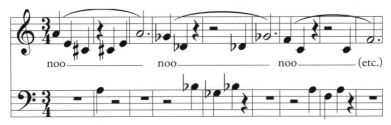

noo_____ noo_____ noo_____ (etc.)

3. Modal to Falsetto, back to Modal Transition

a. For Midvoice II, IIA

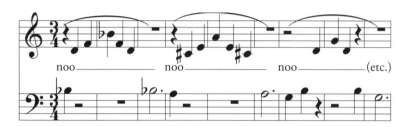

noo———   noo———   noo———   (etc.)

b. For New and Developing Baritones (New/Emerging Adult Voices)

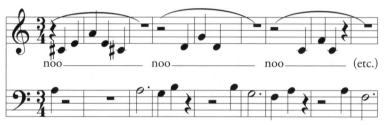

noo———   noo———   noo———   (etc.)

4. Stepwise Patterns: Falsetto to Modal Transition, and Vice Versa

a. For Midvoice II, IIA

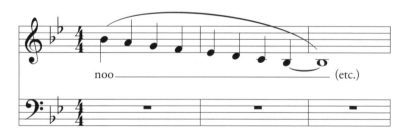

noo———————   (etc.)

Repeat sequence, descending by half steps. Reverse pattern, beginning on B♭3, and go up; repeat sequence by half steps.

b. For New and Developing Baritones

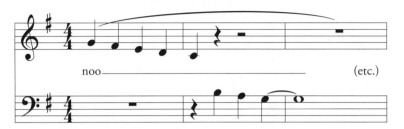

noo⎯⎯⎯⎯⎯⎯⎯⎯⎯⎯⎯⎯⎯⎯⎯⎯⎯⎯⎯⎯⎯⎯ (etc.)

Repeat sequence, descending by half steps. Reverse pattern, beginning on about E3 or F3, and go up. Repeat sequence by half steps.

5. Other Suggestions

a. Use 'whee,' 'hoo,' sliding from falsetto to modal registers, sustaining a final tone in the modal register. Try modal to falsetto, sustaining the final tone in falsetto.

b. Utilize arpeggios, singing from modal to falsetto to modal registers, learning how to use the 'light mechanism,' especially in the passagio region (transition area between modal and falsetto registers). Also employ stepwise, diatonic patterns. The 'oo' vowel is good to use in these exercises.

FULL RANGE UTILIZATION AND RANGE EXTENSION
FOR FEMALE ADOLESCENT VOICES

1.

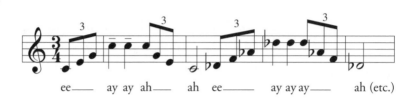

ee——— ay——— ah   ee——— ay——— ah (etc.)

2.

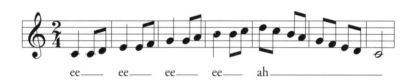

ee——— ay ay ah—— ah   ee——— ay ay ay—— ah (etc.)

3.

ee—— ee—— ee—— ee—— ah————

Ascend by half steps.

Movement Activities

1. Apply knee bends on ascending patterns.

2. Apply circular conducting gestures on the quarter note beat.

3. Apply downward arm motions when the top notes of each exercise are sung.

CHAPTER SIX

SELECTING APPROPRIATE MUSIC FOR CHANGING VOICES

It is very important for the director to select music which matches the ranges and tessituras of voice change stages. This is a difficult but not impossible task. No doubt some compromises will have to be made with published music so that some of these scores can be used with changing voices.

1. Notes can be changed and alternate parts written with the consent of the publisher and/or copyright holder.

2. Voice parts may be assigned to different octaves (e.g.. In three part music, New and Developing Baritones may sing the melody an octave lower).

3. Voices may be assigned to different parts. (e.g. Midvoice II's, and IIA's may sing the third part or lowest voice. In two part music, Midvoice II's/IIA's may sing the alto line.

4. Voices may be assigned to sing only limited sections of the score where ranges are accessible. (e.g. Midvoice II's may join when the refrain of the hymn occurs.)

The *best* solution, however, is to try to find music which *closely matches* the vocal abilities of changing voices. One should consider the following ranges and tessituras when arranging or selecting music for the youth choir.

NOTE: In some cases, when high school singers are also participating, some ranges/tessituras may be a little high for tenors.

A. UNISON MUSIC

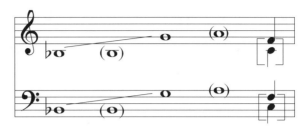

Bracketed notes—tessituras

Composite range for all parts.
Compromises must be made for Midvoice IIA.
Unison tunes in this limited range are hard to find.

B. TWO PART MUSIC

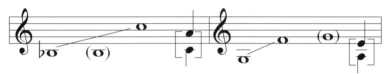

High School Girls	High School Tenors
Unchanged, Midvoice I	Some girls possibly who have lower ranges
Baritones doubling octave lower	Perhaps some Midvoice I's
	Midvoice II, IIA

Bracketed notes—tessituras

C. THREE PART MUSIC

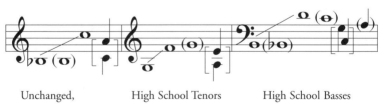

Unchanged,	High School Tenors	High School Basses
Midvoice I	Midvoice II, IIA	New, Developing Baritones
Girls can sing		
either/both Parts I & II		

NOTE: Many 3-part published arrangements contain Baritone parts with the range A3–D3, E3. This is generally too high in terms of tessiturae; however, Midvoice II's, IIA's can sing this quite comfortably. New Voices and Emerging Adult Voices (New Baritone/Settling Baritone) might then possibly sing the top line an octave lower.

D. SATB MUSIC

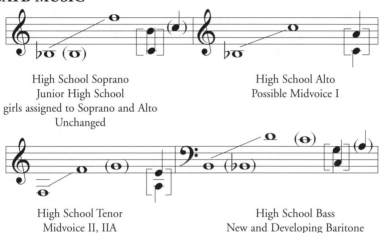

High School Soprano
Junior High School
girls assigned to Soprano and Alto
Unchanged

High School Alto
Possible Midvoice I

High School Tenor
Midvoice II, IIA

High School Bass
New and Developing Baritone

E. TTB MUSIC

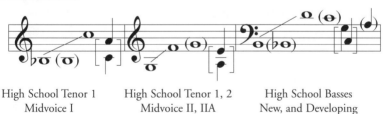

High School Tenor 1
Midvoice I
Unchanged

High School Tenor 1, 2
Midvoice II, IIA

High School Basses
New, and Developing
Baritones

F. TTBB MUSIC

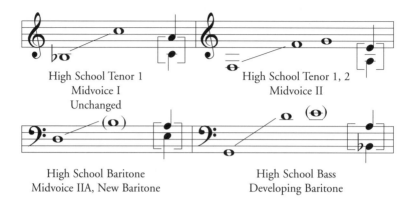

High School Tenor 1
Midvoice I
Unchanged

High School Tenor 1, 2
Midvoice II

High School Baritone
Midvoice IIA, New Baritone

High School Bass
Developing Baritone

There are, of course, other considerations when choosing music for changing voices. The following factors should be taken into account:

1. Avoid music demanding numerous register changes and transitions.

2. Try to find music which will allow students to consolidate the most comfortable area of their singing range first. After this, range extensions (utilizing light mechanism and falsetto techniques) may be attempted. Changing voices are capable of being trained to sing in a wider range (extending from modal to falsetto), but due caution and patience must be exercised. It is best to prominently use the most accessible and comfortable range to prevent poor singing habits (e.g. tight jaw, throat tension, upper body tension, etc...)

3. Be aware of agility requirements. Emerging baritones need special attention in this area. Stepwise movement is much easier than leaps of a fifth, or augmented/diminished intervals. With careful training, these voices can develop more flexibility. It just takes time, patience, and application of good tone production principles.

4. Be aware of the long phrase and its demands. Renaissance music, for example, is often very challenging in this respect.

5. Choose music to meet the breath control capabilities of young adolescents. Brahms and Bach, for example, are often very difficult, but some works by these composers are acceptable. (see Appendix D)

6. Most SSA, SAB music is unsuitable; extensive ranges/tessiturae are prohibiting factors.

7. Avoid trite texts and 'popsy' tunes! Go for quality!

8. Some vocal arrangements should 'spotlight' changing voices. Give them the melody, for example, for one section of the piece.

9. Give singers a VARIETY of music—Renaissance to Contemporary, Folk, etc...

10. Do *not* cater to young peoples' tastes or demands, nor be drawn into the latest musical fads. Choose music which will be challenging, appropriate, appealing, and educationally sound. Young people will appreciate their choral experience more if quality music is presented to them. In the 'long run' a solid foundation for worshipful and artistic communication will be built with this approach.

Choral Arranging

Some choir directors may wish to arrange hymn tunes or other melodies for the changing voice. This is a practical and positive way to encourage young singers to continue their involvement in the choral music program. Music which directly suits their needs will prove to be most rewarding for all concerned.

The following guidelines for arranging were written by Leonard Van Camp, Director of Choral Activities at Southern Illinois University, Edwardsville. Given Dr. Van Camp's background and expertise in the field, these brief, well-chosen comments should be most helpful to those interested in arranging music for the youth choir.

Guidelines

1. Select a limited range melody (6th to an octave).

2. Carefully select the key that will keep the melody in the range of the changing voices.

3. Give the melody to the changing voices much of the time.

4. Assess the musicianship of each voice part in the choir and tailor a part to help them feel successful.

5. Keep it simple. Consider the time needed to learn each phrase. Is a 'fancy idea' worth the time to teach it?

6. Use repeated or ostinato ideas when possible.

7. Write out the ranges and tessiturae you intend to observe on each line of the staff paper.

8. Consider: breath capacity, easy intervals and good voice leading, ease of finding initial pitches after rests, vowels used on high pitches, the need for each part to rest, and the need for alternate pitches in some lines.

9. Type the words out first and space the manuscript carefully. Make clear, legible notation to save valuable rehearsal time.

10. Consider the arrangement an experiment, and be prepared to go 'back to the drawing board' after hearing it.

Music well-selected and/or arranged forms the backbone of the youth choir program. If the special needs of the changing voice are met, young singers will be more encouraged to stay in the program and continue lifelong participation in singing. Appendix C contains a 'selective' sample of music which has been performed most effectively by Junior High School and Church Youth Choirs.

CLOSING COMMENTS

The youth choir director's sensitivity to the vocal needs of changing adolescent male and female singers will help to enhance all aspects of the church youth music program. Young people will sing better, maintain a healthier attitude about themselves as individuals, gain confidence in performing, and contribute constructively to the development of a truly comprehensive music program of the church. By being able to 'sing through the change,' young men especially will stand a better chance of remaining involved with music through the high school years and beyond. It is vitally important, as has been stressed throughout this publication, that choir directors first understand the maturation process. While dealing with the various stages can be somewhat complicated at times, the end result is well worth the effort. Voice classification is a key ingredient, and can be accomplished on a group or individual basis. After this has been done, the choir director is ready to apply principles of good tone production and kinesthetics in the choral rehearsal; furthermore, he or she will know how to exercise the male and female voice during the different maturational stages so that good tone quality, resonance, intervallic-rhythmic vocal agility, and smooth register transitions can be achieved. By wisely selecting and/or arranging choral music appropriate to the range abilities of changing voices, effective performance will result. This also allows voice development to proceed on a natural course, without interruption or undue stress. In short, the youth choir has the potential to achieve outstanding results if these factors are taken into account. Increased understanding of adolescent voice change and implementation of appropriate methodologies provides the solid foundation and right formula for success and continued development of the church youth music program.

APPENDIX A

SUMMARY OF THE STAGES OF VOICE MATURATION IN THE ADOLESCENT MALE

Premutation Stage: Unchanged Voice Classification

A. **AGE:** Height of pre-pubertal period. Unchanged voice reaches climax of beauty and 'fullness.' Optimum period: Grade 5 to Grade 6. Sometimes to early Grade 7. Age span: usually 10–11 years of age.

B. **VOICE DURING SPEECH:** Average Speaking Fundamental Frequency (SFF) A3 to C4 in the majority of cases. 'Light' voice quality.

C. **VOICE DURING SINGING:** Full, rich soprano-like quality. Reaches its pinnacle of beauty, power and intensity during this time. Range expansion of the childhood voice at its maximum. Breaks/shifts caused by inappropriate application of heavy mechanism in lower register. Typically boys may sing too heavily in the lower range, and therefore shift quite noticeably when going to higher pitches. Average range is A3–F5; tessitura is C#4–A4.

D. **ACOUSTICS:** Retains full spectrum of overtones in each tone. Upper partial range (4100–8000Hz) not yet affected by maturation. Full array of upper frequency amplitudes. Average of 2–3 formants in lower partial range (80–4100Hz), and two for the upper partial range. Dynamic range approaches healthy adult norms.

E. **PHYSIOLOGICAL:** Pre-pubertal; therefore growth spurt not yet started. Some 'baby' fat on body frame.

F. **PART ASSIGNMENT:** Usually sings soprano part, but also capable of singing Soprano II or Alto. Can easily sing in A3 to F5 pitch range.

G. **AGILITY:** Very flexible, agile voice with good capability for dynamic variation.

Early Mutation Stage: Midvoice I Classification

A. **AGE:** Initial pubertal period. Lasts from 1 to 5 months on the average but can extend to 12 months or more. Can begin in Grade 6; majority in Grade 7, between ages of 12 and 13. Some may begin this stage as late as the eighth grade. The onset of pubertal sexual and voice development can not be predicted with any degree of precision.

B. **VOICE DURING SPEECH:** Average Speaking Fundamental Frequency (SFF) A3–B3 in the majority of cases. Light voice quality. Very little perceptual change from the Unchanged period. Sometimes breathier tone, especially above C5.

C. **VOICE DURING SINGING:** Variable loss of tonal clarity and 'richness' in higher pitches, most notably in the C5–F5 range, but there is a noticeable increase in breathiness and constriction especially in upper pitch extremes. Pitches can initially be sounded in the C5–F5 range, but there is a noticeable increase in breathiness and constriction. Generally, tone quality is thinner and not as rich in harmonic partials in that range. In the Cooksey, et al., study, subjects' average ranges decreased from 20.6 semitones in the Unchanged classification to 16.6 semitones in the Midvoice I Classification. Average tessitura ranges decreased from 9.1 semitones to 8.1 semitones.

D. **ACOUSTICS:** There is a decrease in perceptual 'richness' of the tone. Generally, higher frequency formants are decreasing in amplitude in the lower and upper pitches of modal register. Lower frequency formant amplitudes remain stable. Both gross vocal volume and singing dynamic range are constant, still approaching healthy adult norms.

E. **PHYSIOLOGICAL:** Hormone secretions begin to trigger many physical changes, such as an increase in the amount of body fat, height and weight. The vocal folds begin to lengthen and thicken. Laryngeal cartilage structure begins to grow larger and change configuration, and muscles increase in size. Secondary sexual development begins and the first appearance of pubic hair occurs. Most of these changes are just beginning and are somewhat subtle in this stage. The Cooksey, et al., study showed strong increases, however, in total body fat, vital capacity, and weight.

F. **PART ASSIGNMENT:** Usually sings alto part in SATB music, but still has the most desirable vocal 'color' and 'power' in the mid-range area, D4–B4/C5. Sometimes, SATB alto parts too low and the soprano part is too high. Optimum pitch range is A♭3–C5.

G. **AGILTY:** Not as flexible or agile in upper range because of increasing size of vocal folds.

High Mutation Stage: Midvoice II Classification

A. **AGE:** This stage is the height of mutational change. Normal age is 13–14 years, but there are many exceptions. Midvoice II's can be found in 6th grade and sometimes 5th grade. A majority of boys have passed through this stage by the Spring of 9th grade. In the Cooksey, et al., study, the average time boys spent in Midvoice II was 12–13 months. There was, however, a large variance, ranging from 2 months to 19 months. A majority of boys in this classification were found in grades 7–8, with the largest percentage found during Spring of the 7th grade year to Winter of the 8th grade year.

B. **VOICE DURING SPEECH:** Average SFF is lower and easily perceived when compared to the Unchanged classification. Voice quality for Midvoice II is noticeably 'huskier,' 'thicker,' and sometimes 'breathy.' It is not as 'light' as Midvoice I. Eighty-four per cent of the subjects in the Cooksey, et al., study had average SFF's between G3–A♯3, with the majority at about G♯3–A3. Beginning with this stage, the average SFF became stabilized at 3 to 4 semitones above the Low Terminal Pitch (LTP) of the singing range.

C. **VOICE DURING SINGING:** This classification produces a unique voice quality that is 'huskier' and 'thicker' than Midvoice I, evidenced by an increase in noise levels in the upper partial range (4100–8000Hz). Voices do not have the 'richness' and 'fullness' of adult-like tone. Amplitude of spectral partials is much weaker when compared to the premutational stage. In the Cooksey, et al., study, pitch range decreased slightly to 15.5 semitones, but the range of tessiturae remained about the same as Midvoice I. Higher modal pitches were extremely unstable. The transition zone (passagio) between modal and falsetto registers was F4–C5. Falsetto and whistle registers emerged. Falsetto began at G4–D5, with the majority beginning at about A4. The maturation process has increased the instability of vocal coordination, particularly in regard to upper pitch range accuracy. There is stability in the lower pitch range.

D. **ACOUSTICS:** A decrease continued in upper partial range formant energy (amplitude/intensity) when the boys sustained lower and upper modal register pitches. There were further increases in noise components for this stage. When compared to Midvoice I, noise levels of Midvoice II's almost doubled in their lower partial range (80–4,000Hz) when the boys sang lower and upper pitches in modal register. Falsetto register was relatively free from constriction effects. Gross volume and singing dynamic range increased slightly and continued to approximate healthy adult norms.

E. **PHYSIOLOGICAL:** The 'shield' of the larynx, the thyroid cartilage, becomes more sharply angled, creating a relatively prominent, protruding 'Adams Apple.' Bodily height, chest size, vital capacity, and weight continue to increase. There is a slight decrease in percentage of body fat. Many boys show disparities in body proportions. Maximum development now is occurring in primary/secondary sexual characteristics. There are increases in the average amount of phonation time. In the Cooksey, et al., study, phonation quotient was lowest of all the stages, indicating increased efficiency in vocal fold approximation. Subjects produced surprising gross volume capabilities and this was reflected in increases in singing dynamic range measurements.

F. **PART ASSIGNMENT:** Skill in vocal part assignment by teachers and conductors is crucial for boys in this classification. Alto parts often are too high; tenor parts too low. Optimum pitch area is F3–F4/G4.

G. **AGILITY:** Midvoice II's are not as agile when compared to unchanged voices. Avoiding the upper pitch area (the most unstable part of their range), will help them avoid future hyperfunction, until healthy, efficient singing coordinations are established. Range extension then may be possible by using the falsetto register to learn how to 'melt' the register transitions. If boys produce the falsetto register with excess effort, then use of the falsetto technique should be avoided or delayed until natural register coordinations develop.

Mutational Climax Stage: Midvoice IIA Classification

A. **AGE:** This stage of voice change coincides with the climactic period of puberty. In the Cooksey, et al., study, Midvoice IIA lasted an average of 4 to 5 months, but varied between 3 weeks to 10 months—even longer in a few cases. A majority of the boys in this classification were in the 8th grade. A significant upsurge occurred, however, in the final month of the 7th grade. There was a sharp decline in the number of Midvoice IIA's in the 9th grade. The normal age span of boys for Midvoice IIA was 13–14 years of age, with a mean age of 13.6.

B. **VOICE DURING SPEECH:** In the Cooksey, et al., study, the majority of average SFF's occurred at F3–F♯3. Voice quality is 'huskier,' 'thicker' than Midvoice II, perhaps perceptually 'thinner sounding.' These voices are very susceptible to hoarseness and abuse. Register 'breaks' are very apparent during this time.

C. **VOICE DURING SINGING:** High Terminal and Low Terminal Pitches are lower than Midvoice II, although the range span is about the same. There is extreme instability in the upper pitch range where strain can occur easily. Perceptually, listeners can hear some of the emerging baritone quality in the lower pitch range, but the upper range remains light and often displays increased breathiness and strain. There is a very common tendency toward hyperfunction, or 'pushing' and the use of 'heavy mechanism' during this stage. Transition to falsetto can be extremely difficult, with some voices not able to sing in that register at all. Due to changes in musculature of the larynx (and some muscle weakness in the arytenoid area), the whistle register becomes more prominent. Singers often have perceptual difficulties in matching pitch at times. Part of this can be due to placement in the choir and confusion on the part of the teacher in assigning the voice to its appropriate pitch range.

In the Cooksey, et al., study, the extent of pitch and tessitura ranges remained about equal to Midvoice II. High Terminal Pitches and Low Terminal Pitches of their ranges were lower. A majority of subjects showed register 'lift points' between E4 and B4, but half the subjects changed to falsetto register on G4. The most problematic transition area for registers was D4–G4. Average pitch range was D3–F♯4, and tessitura range was F♯3 to C4/D4/E4.

D. **ACOUSTICS:** Noise and amplitude level statistics showed that this is the weakest, most vulnerable voice maturation stage. By this time, constriction resulting from intrinsic laryngeal muscle strain was evident in many of the lower range partials. General noise levels increased in lower partial range (80–4000Hz) of modal register, and this trend continued in succeeding voice classifications. This data indicated a decreased energy (amplitude/intensity) throughout the singing range. There was a slight increase in gross volume and singing dynamic range.

E. **PHYSIOLOGICAL:** In the Cooksey, et al., study, there were dramatic increases in weight, and steady increases in height, chest size, waist size, and vital capacity. Body fat percentages continued to decline. Sustained phonation time increased. Maximal development of primary/secondary sexual characteristics occurred. There was decreased vocal fold oscillation efficiency.

F. **PART ASSIGNMENT:** This is the most problematic classification for part assignment. Most published music is unsuitable. Optimum pitch range for singing is F3–D4.

G. **AGILITY:** Voice is weaker, less flexible, and a moderate pitch range for singing would be helpful for voice skill development. An emphasis on release of unnecessary neck-throat muscles and efficient laryngeal coordination is needed. Cultivation of easy phonation will be valuable. Be cautious in the use of falsetto register.

Postmutational Stabilizing Stage:
New Baritone/New Voice Classification

[Please note that in these classification guidelines, the term 'baritone' is chosen as a matter of convenience. Be mindful of the additional terminology—"New Voice" and/or "Emerging Adult Voice" when referring to this classification. The terminology does not imply adult baritone characteristics.]

A. **AGE:** This classification represents the end of the most dramatic stage of voice change. Many aspects of mutational processes are stabilizing. In the Cooksey, et al., study, the New Baritone/New Voice designation lasted an average of 3–5 months, but varied between 4 weeks and 8 months. A significant upsurge occurred in the number of boys in this classification during the last few months of 7th grade. An even more dramatic upsurge occurred over the summer months between 7th and 8th grades. There was a large percentage of boys in this classification in the 8th and 9th grades. Normal mean age was approximately 14 years, but varied beween 13–15 years of age.

B. **VOICE DURING SPEECH:** In the Cooksey, et al., study, a majority of the average SFF's occurred between C3–E3. Lower pitches were quite evident. Quality was 'thin,' and 'light,' compared to adult quality. Voice quality was more consistently alike across individuals, (e.g.,unique individual characterisics were not very prominent.)

78

C. **VOICE DURING SINGING:** The New Baritone/New Voice voice quality can be very firm and clear, but continues to sound 'immature,' 'light,' 'thin,' and lacking in the 'richness' of a typical adult male voice. There is less breathiness and constriction, generally. There is very little vibrato. Some listeners may 'hear' this voice an octave higher than it actually is, and some listeners may hear it an octave lower than it is. Usually, there is a much more stable transition area between modal and falsetto registers. Falsetto register begins to stabilize in a majority of voices beginning around D4–E4. The general transition area at C4–F4 is difficult for some singers. During this classification, the voices of some boys may be able to sing reasonably well in their lower range, but as they attempt to sing toward a higher range, their falsetto register may 'pop in' at G4, having skipped a number of pitches in between. This 'blank spot' is not uncommon. With further maturation and guided experience over time, those pitches return. Appropriate and helpful vocalises that utilize falsetto register to 'lighten' their upper range modal register sometimes enable a 'return' of the 'missing' pitches.

In the Cooksey, et al., study, the extent of pitch range equaled Midvoice IIA (15.5 semitones), but tessitura range decreased to 7.4 semitones (Midvoice IIA was 8.1). Voices were much more stable and consistent throughout the modal range, and falsetto register pitches became easier to produce.

D. **ACOUSTICS:** In the Cooksey, et al., study, there was still no sign of a return of amplitude 'strength' in upper frequency partials for lower and upper sustained pitches in modal register, as revealed in sonagraphs of the subjects in this voice classification. These acoustic measures indicate the first emergence toward normal adult data, but still do not have the numerous harmonic partials and formant regions typical of the adult male voice. Gross volume and singing dynamic range remained unchanged from the previous stage.

E. **PHYSIOLOGICAL:** In the Cooksey, et al., study, increases in height, weight, chest size, and vital capacity continued, with a generally correlated decrease in percentage of body fat. There was a slight decrease in the duration of phonation on a single inhalation/exhalation. The phonation quotient was much higher indicating decreased vocal fold ocscillation efficiency. That characteristic is normal for voices with emerging register differentiations, and also indicates that maturity has not yet been achieved in changing voices.

F. **PART ASSIGNMENT:** Many bass parts are too low. Optimum range for singing is B♭2 to C4–D4.

G. **AGILITY:** Lacks agility, flexibility, and often becomes heavy when *fortissimo* dynamics are called for. Frequent 'flatting' occurs when the voice is 'overworked.' Cultivation of 'lighter mechanism' and efficient breath energy in singing will enable increased agility.

Postmutational Development Stage:
Developing Baritone/Emerging Adult Voice Classification

A. **AGE:** This stage represents a marked tendency toward vocal maturity, and the emergence of a young man's personal vocal 'signature.' Adult-like characteristics still are not apparent, but unique voice qualities begin to appear. This stage is a period of gradual range expansion and growth in vocal anatomy. The Developing Baritone/Emerging Adult Voice Classification is prominent among 9th grade boys, and begins generally at 14–15 years of age.

B. **VOICE DURING SPEECH:** The majority of average SFF's now occur between A2–C♯3, with the average at B2. Thicker, heavier voice quality is now apparent. Generally speaking there is more stability and consistency in voice production. Low Terminal Pitch, in some cases, is 'distancing itself' from the average SFF. In some cases Low Terminal Pitch may be as much as 4–6 semitones lower than the average SFF.

C. **VOICE DURING SINGING:** The trend established in the New Baritone/New Voice stage continues, with quality becoming more clear and 'focused,' but still lacking in the greater richness associated with adult voices. Voices at this age are not physically mature enough to produce the tone qualities, ranges,e etc..., that the adult categories of tenor, bass, and baritone can produce. Note also that there is still little vibrato developing during this time, although unique resonance characteristics are beginning to appear. Falsetto register is very clear and 'focused.' The register transition area is slightly lower than New Baritone/New Voice, but the majority of boys will begin falsetto register at D3–E3. Upper range passagio area is C4–F4. Upper and falsetto registers are easier to manage now. In the Cooksey, et al., study, pitch range began to expand rather significantly, from 15.5 semitones for New Baritones/New Voices to 19.2 semitones. Tessitura range also expanded from 7.4 semitones for New Baritones/New Voices to 8.2 semitones for Developing Baritones/Emerging Adult Voices.

D. **ACOUSTICS:** Noise in the lower partial range (80–4000Hz) continues to increase when boys sustain a lower pitch in modal register, but that lower partial range noise decreases when boys sustain a higher pitch in modal register. Noise in the lower partial range decreases in falsetto register. Phonation patterns are still somewhat erratic and motor control is still not secure. Overall harmonic energy (amplitude) still does not approach adult norms or match those found in the unchanged voice. The means of center of upper level formants in the upper partial range (as displayed by a lower pitch in modal register) remain about even with the New Baritone/New Voice classification. There is an increase in the means of centers of upper level formants when boys are sustaining a higher pitch in modal register. The first and second average formant locations continue to decrease, indicating increased size of the vocal tract from physical growth, but they still do not approximate adult norms. Gross volume and singing dynamic ranges increase slightly.

E. **PHYSIOLOGICAL:** There is dense growth of pubic and auxilliary hair in body development. Chest and shoulder dimensions continue to increase, as does weight, height, and vital capacity. A dramatic increase in weight occurs, but percentage of body fat remains stable. Vocal folds have reached maximum length, and vocal tract cavities are approaching completed size and configuration. There is a strong increase in phonation quotient indicating weaker glottal efficiency. Apparently, voices in this stage still must develop much more before adult norms can be matched.

F. **PART ASSIGNMENT:** Can sing most bass parts; some may sing high baritone. Optimum pitch area: B♭2–A3.

G. **AGILITY:** Greater agility when compared to New Baritone/New Voices, but physical development and 'motor brain programming' must continue before adult agility can be approached. More flexibility is available in the upper pitch range area and in transitions to falsetto register. Again, cultivate the 'lighter mechanism' for modal/falsetto singing. Many boys still will have a tendency to 'push.'

APPENDIX B

SUMMARY OF THE STAGES OF VOICE MATURATION IN THE ADOLESCENT FEMALE*

Prepubertal

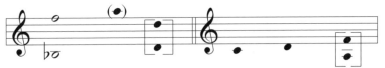

Pitch Range for Lower and Upper Registers

Bracketed notes—tessituras

Average Speaking Fundamental Frequency and Wilson's Acceptable Limits

A. **AGE:** 8–10/11 years of age. Depending on other physiological changes, such as breast development and menarche, this stage could continue through age 12 or 13 years.

B. **VOICE DURING SPEECH:** Average fundamental frequency is C4–D4; **acceptable limits: A3–F4.

C. **VOICE DURING SINGING:** Light, flute-like, child soprano quality; no apparent register 'breaks;' flexible, able to manage intervallic skips; much like male voices at the same age with the exception that female voices are lighter in 'weight' because the volume potential is generally not as great.

*Copied with permission from *Bodymind and Voice,* Thurman, L. and Welch, G. eds., Book 5, Chapter 7: "Female Adolescent Changing Voices: Voice Classification, Voice Skill Development, and Music Literature Selection," Lynne Gackle, 583–84.

**Voice Problems of Children,* Wilson, D.K. Baltimore, MD: Williams and Wilkins, 1987, 116–24.

Pubescence/Pre-Menarcheal

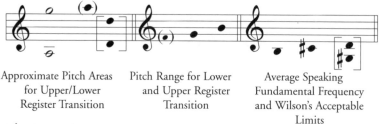

| Approximate Pitch Areas for Upper/Lower Register Transition | Pitch Range for Lower and Upper Register Transition | Average Speaking Fundamental Frequency and Wilson's Acceptable Limits |

Bracketed notes—tessituras

A. **AGE:** Beginning of Mutation, Ages 11–12/13; first signs of physical maturation, such as breast development, height increase, etc...

B. **VOICE DURING SPEECH:** Average fundamental frequency is B3–C♯4; **acceptable limits: A♯3–D4.

C. **VOICE DURING SINGING:** Breathiness in the tone due to appearance of mutational 'chink,' an inadequate closure of the vocal folds as growth occurs in the laryngeal area. Register transition or 'break' typically appears between G4 and B4; sometimes, an apparent loss of lower pitch range occurs around C4. (Some girls have trouble producing the lower register at this time.)

D. **SIGNS:** Singing becomes difficult, and at times, is uncomfortable; difficulty in achieving desired volume (especially in the middle and upper range); breathy voice quality throughout the pitch range. Because of increased vocal fold dimensions, voice quality becomes 'thicker' or 'weightier.'

Puberty/Post-Menarcheal

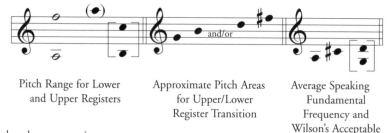

| Pitch Range for Lower and Upper Registers | Approximate Pitch Areas for Upper/Lower Register Transition | Average Speaking Fundamental Frequency and Wilson's Acceptable Limits |

Bracketed notes—tessituras

A. **AGE:** Peak of mutation, Ages 13–14/15

B. **VOICE DURING SPEECH:** Average fundamental frequency is A3–C♯4; **acceptable limits: G3–D4.

C. **VOICE DURING SINGING:** Very critical time. After Stage IIA (Pre-menarcheal), tessitura can move up or down, or sometimes, can narrow at either end, yielding a basic six or seven note range of 'comfortable singing;' register breaks still apparent between G4 and B4, and also at D5–F♯5. At times, lower register pitch range is more easily produced yielding an illusion of an 'alto' quality; singing in this range may be easier and can be recommended for short periods of time. (Note: Singing only in the lower range for an indefinite period of time may be injurious to a young 'unsettled' voice because of a tendency to sing and speak in lower register with excessive larynx and vocal tract constriction, resulting in excessive vocal fold impact and shear forces and possible voice disorders.) Vocalization throughout the vocal pitch range will help development of lengthener-prominent larynx coordinations, and aid in overall vocal fold conditioning by stretching them to increase tissue compliance and agility; avoiding any unnecessary effort and constriction in the lower or upper range will aid the process of learning physically efficient voice skills. Because the changes during this stage are sporadic and unpredictable, it is necessary to listen to individual voices frequently in order to assess vocal development.

D. **SIGNS:** Hoarseness without upper respiratory infection; voice 'cracking;' singing is difficult (especially in the upper pitch range), and at times, uncomfortable. Some breathiness and lack of clarity in the tone. Often, voice quality is more full-bodied in the lower register, with a relatively abrupt 'flip' into a breathy, more child-like, 'flutey' voice quality when transitioning from lower to upper registers.

Young Adult Female/Post-Menarcheal

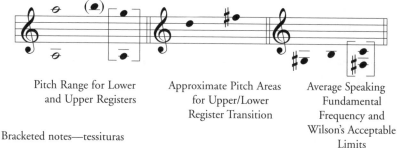

Pitch Range for Lower
and Upper Registers

Bracketed notes—tessituras

Approximate Pitch Areas
for Upper/Lower
Register Transition

Average Speaking
Fundamental
Frequency and
Wilson's Acceptable
Limits

A. **AGE:** Settling and developing toward adult capabilities, 14–15/16 years of age.

B. **VOICE DURING SPEECH:** Average fundamental frequency is G♯3–B3; acceptable limits: F♯3–C4. Timbre approximates that of an adult female; more 'full-bodied richness' appears in voice quality.

C. **VOICE DURING SINGING:** Overall pitch and volume range capabilities increase. (In some girls pitch range does not appear to lower during the time of voice mutation. One characteristic of skilled singing, however, is a developed ability to sing a wide range of pitches—lower to higher. Simply because a young singer can sing with a full-bodied voice quality in lower register does not imply that the singer is an alto.) Breathiness appears to decrease and there is more consistency of tonal quality between upper and lower registers; register 'breaks' are more common at the secondo passaggio D5–F♯5 (more typical of female adult voices). Voice quality is more full-bodied, richer, and fuller, though not as much as a mature adult. More ease returns in singing coordinations. Vibrato may appear, and vocal agility increases.

Appendix C

Individual Audition Form

Name _____ Date _____

Address _____ Grade _____

Parent's Name _____ Telephone _____

Choir_____

Previous Experience in Music

_____

_____

Do you play the piano? _____If so, for how long? _____

Do you play another instrument? _____How long: _____

Voice Evaluation

*Key: 1-2, low;   3-5, Medium/normal;   6-8, High

Matching tones	1 2 3 4 5 6 7 8
Sense of rhythm	1 2 3 4 5 6 7 8
Tonal memory	1 2 3 4 5 6 7 8
Degree of breathiness	1 2 3 4 5 6 7 8
Degree of constriction	1 2 3 4 5 6 7 8
Degree of Pitch agility	1 2 3 4 5 6 7 8
Breath support	1 2 3 4 5 6 7 8
Posture	1 2 3 4 5 6 7 8
Diction	1 2 3 4 5 6 7 8
Volume	1 2 3 4 5 6 7 8

Range and Tessitura: Voice Classification_____

_____

_____

_____

APPENDIX D

CHORAL MUSIC FOR ADOLESCENT CHANGING VOICES

Music for Male Ensembles

"Beautiful Savior," Butler, Jack (Arr.), TTBB, Willis Music Co., Cincinnati, OH, W9782.

"Boatmen Stomp," Gray, Michael, Three Parts, Morris Hayes Series, G. Schirmer, 12396.

"Children Go Where I Send Thee," Crocker, Emily, TTB. Jenson Pub., 471-03041.

"Climbin' Up the Mountain," Smith, W.H., (Arr.), TTBB, Neil A. Kjos Pub., Ed. 1101.

"De Animals a-comin," Bartholomew, (Arr.), TTBB, G. Schirmer, 8946.

"Good News," Brown, Gary, TTB, *Enter the Young Series,* Studio Pub., Hialeah, FL, V 7707-3.

"Integer Vitae," Flemming/Johnstone, CCBB, Cambiata Press, M97562.

"O, What Joy that I Have Jesus" ("Jesu, Joy of Man's Desiring"), Bach, J.S., Van Camp, Leonard (Arr.), Male voices in three choirs, Southern Music Co., San Antonio, Tx, SC 325.

"Kyrie," Krunnfusz, Dan, TB, Pentref Publications, Box 78, Baraboo, WI 53913, 2B-8803.

"Lo, How a Rose e'er Blooming," Praetorius, M., TTBB, E.C. Schirmer, 24.

"Masters in this Hall," Chartres, Burger, D., (Arr.), TBB, Studio Pub., Columbia Pictures, Hialeah, FL, SV8221.

"Now Thank We All Our God," Cain, N. (Arr.), TTB, Shawnee Press (Flammer Press), C-5028.

"Promised Land," Richardson, M. (Arr.), TTBB, Mark Foster, MF 1005.

"Ride the Chariot," Smith, (Arr.), TTBB, Neil A. Kjos Music Co., 1102.

"Sing We the Praise of God," Bach, J.S. (from Cantata 142), TTBB, Ed. E. Coggin, G. Schirmer, 11471.

"The Sky Can Still Remember," Gray, M. SAB (Morris Hayes Series), G. Schirmer, 12442, SAB.

"Verdant Meadows," Handel, G.F., Gibb, R.W., (Arr.), TTBB, Belwin Mills, F.E.C., 9249.

Selections for Mixed Chorus

"Adoramus Te," (Ed.,) Clement/Clemens non Papa, SATB, (possible for TTBB), N. Greyson, Bourne Co., B200048-358.

"Alleluia! Sing Praise," Bach, J.S., C. Hirt, (Ed.), SATB, C. Fischer, CM7140.

"A Psalm of Assurance," Butler, E., SATB, Hinshaw Music, HMC-175.

"Calypso Noel," Krunnfusz, G., SATB (Variable Voicing), Shawnee Press, A-884.

"Cantate Domino," (Ed.), Pitoni, SATB, N. Greyson, Bourne Co., ES 5.

"Carlos Dominquez," Ades, (Arr.), SATB, Shawnee Press, A-1208.

"Consecrate the Place and Day," Pfautsch, Lloyd, SATB, Lawson-Gould/G. Schirmer, 51420.

"Da Pacem Domine," Franck, Goetze, Mary, (Arr.), Four Equal Parts, Boosey and Hawkes, 6187.

"Dormi, Dormi," Goetze, Mary, (Arr.), Unison, Boosey and Hawkes, 6128.

"Enatus est Emmanuel," Praetorius, M., SATB, Concordia Pub., 98-1868.

"Ev'ry Time I Feel the Spirit," Dawson, (Arr.), SATB, Tuskegee-Kjos, T117.

"Ev'ry Time I Feel the Spirit," Thygerson, R.W., (Arr.), Two Parts Heritage Music Press, H5702.

"Exsultate Justi," Perry, Dave and Jean, SSATB(B), Studio Publications, SV9661.

"Follow the Drinkin' Gourd," Bray, Julie Gardner, SATB, Heritage Choral Series, 15/1116.

"Gloria in excelsis Deo," Vivaldi, A., Thomas, E., (Ed.), SATB, Roger Dean Pub. Co., HRD 183.

"Goin' Up to Glory," Thomas, Andre, SATB, Heritage Choral Series, 15/1228H.

"Gonna Build a Mountain," Leyden, (Arr.), SATB, TRO-Richmond Org., S7011.

"Hallelujah, Amen," (from *Judas Maccabaeus*), Handel, G.F., Brooks, Byron, (Ed.), SATB, Plymouth Music Co., CC7.

"How Excellent Thy Name," Handel, G.F., Herrmann, (Ed.), SATB, G. Schirmer, 11106, 2-piano acc.

"I Will Sing Praises," Booker/Thomas, SATB, Chorister's Guild/Lorenz Corp., CGA718.

"I Will Sing the Goodness of the Lord," Crocker, Emily SATB, Jeenson Pub., 471-09024.

"If Ye Would Hear the Angels Sing," Butt, James, (Arr.), Unison, Boosey and Hawkes, 5566.

"Keep Your Lamps!" Thomas, Andre (Arr.), SATB, Mark Foster Music Co., MF 261.

"Kyrie Eleison," Butler, E., Three-part Mixed, Carl Fischer, CM 8177.

"Lord, I Trust Thee," Handel, G.F., Darlow, Denys, (Ed.), SATB, Oxford Univ. Press, E110.

"Lord of the Dance," Carter, Sydney, Willcocks, David, (Arr.) SSATB, Hope Publishing Co. (The Fourth Presbyterian Church of Chicago Anthem Series), FPC 136.

"Mary, Mary," Avery and Marsh, Jennings, C., (Arr.) SATB, Curtis Music Press, C7943.

"My Lord," Eilers, J. Three-parts, Hal Leonard, 08545500.

"Non e tempo," Cara, M., (from *Three Frottola*), Sturm, G., (Ed.), SATB, European American Music Corporation, EA 119.

"Now Thank We All Our God," Bach, J.S., Haberlen, John, (Ed.), SATB, Neil Kjos, Jr., San Diego, CA, Ed 5975.

"O Come, All Ye Faithful," Dello Joio, N., SATB, E.B. Marks, 15604-8, 4-hand piano.

"O Praise the Lord," Graun, Karl H., Cramer, J., (Ed.), SATB, Marks/Belwin Mills, 4281.

"Popule Meus," Victoria, SATB, Associated Music Pub., A419.

"Psallite," Praetorius, M., Greyson, N., (Ed.), SATB, Bourne, B210658-358.

"Psalm 100 (Jubilate Deo)," Roth, R. N., Unison, E.C. Kerby Ltd., Toronto, 198 Davenport Road, Ontario, Canada, 81071-924.

"Sing a New Song to the Lord," Hopson, Hal, Unison, Choristers Guild, P.O. Box 38188, Dallas, Tx. 75238, A-204.

"Siyahamba," African Song, SATB, Boosey and Hawkes, OCTB6564.

"Speak to One Another of Psalms," Berger, Jean, SATB, Augsburg Fortress Press, 954.

"The Sky Can Still Remember," Gray, M., SAB, (Morris Hayes Series), G. Schirmer, 12442.

"There Is Music in My Soul," Lightfoot, Mary Lynn, SATB, Raymond A. Hoffman Co., H5013.

"When the Trumpet Sounds," Thomas, Andre, SATB, Mark Foster Music Co., MF 261.

"Young King," Harris, Ed, 3-parts, Jenson Publications, 416-25010.

Selections for Treble Chorus

"A Carroll," Jacobson, Betty, SSA, Summy-Birchard Co., B-965.

"A Child is Born," Page, Nick, SSAA, Boosey and Hawkes, OCTB6762.

"A Christmas Lullaby," Vaughan, Rodger, Unison, H. Flammer, F-5001.

"Ave Verum," Faure, G., 2 parts, Roger Dean Pub. Co., HCE-114.

"Babe of Beauty," Boda, John, Unison, Concordia Pub. House, 98-1656.

"Be Like the Bird," Frackenpohl, Arthur, SA, Neil A. Kjos Jr., Pub., Ed. 6118.

"Christmas Dance of the Shepherds," Kodaly, Z., SA, Universal Pub., UE 10878.

"Come to Bethlehem," Warlock, P., SA, G. Schirmer, 10751.

"Corpus Christi Carol," Britten, B., Unison, Oxford Pub., E94.

"Da Pacem Domine," Goetze, Mary, 4 part treble, Boosey and Hawkes, OCTB6187.

"Dormi, Dormi," Goetze, Mary, Unison, Boosey and Hawkes, OCTB6128.

"Eucaristica, (Deep in my heart I bear my Lord)," Casals, P., Three-part treble, Tetra Music Corp./A. Broude, A.B. 155-5.

"Fancie," Britten, B., Unison, Boosey and Hawkes, 5611.

"Father William," Fine, Irving, SSA, Warner Bros.Pub., 2-w3204.

"Gloria in Excelsis Deo," Pierce, B., SA, Plymouth Music Co., Inc., BP-503.

"Hashivenu," Rao, Canon, Boosey and Hawkes, OC3B6430.

"Hodie," de Caelo, Nobis, Grandi, A., SA, Mark Foster Co., MF 803.

"How Brightly Shines the Morning Star," Praetorius, M., SA, Boosey and Hawkes, OCTB6419.

"I Sing of a Maiden," Hadleu, P., Two-part treble, Ascherberg, Hopwood and Crew, Ltd.(Royal School of Church Music), No. 265.

"I'm Goin' Home on a Cloud," Tatlor-Howell, Susan, Four-part treble, Boosey and Hawkes, OCTB6389.

"In the Highlands," Butler, SSA, Carl Fischer, CM7852.

"Joyfully We Go Now to Bethlehem," Schutz, H., SSA, Pro Art/Belwin Mills, PROCH 3022.

"Jubilate Deo," Praetorius, M., Rao, D., (Arr.), Four-part treble, Boosey and Hawkes, OCTB6350.

"King Herod and the Cock," Britten, B., (Arr.), Unison, Boosey and Hawkes, 5612.

"Like as the Father," Cherubini, L., Three Equal Voices, Summy-Birchard, 5297.

"Long, Long Ago," Floyd, C., Two parts, Boosey and Hawkes, 5648.

"Lovely Child, Holy Child," Johnson, D., (Arr.), SAA, Augsburg Fortress Press, CS 526.

"Lullaby," Vaughan Williams, R., SA, Oxford University Press, 44.603.

"Lullay my liking," Holst, G., SSAA, G. Schirmer, 11750.

"Nigra Sum," Casals, P,. Two-parts, Alexander Broude, 120-8.

"Nova, Nova, Ave Fit Ex Eva," Spencer, W., SSA, National Music Pub., WHCC 14.

"On Christmas Night," Vaughan Williams, R., Unison, Galaxy Music. Pub., 337.

"Rise Up, My Love, My Fair One," McCray, J., SSA, National Music Pub., WHC-44.

Sleep Little One," Nelson, R., SSA, Boosey and Hawkes, 5262.

"Sound the Trumpet," Purcell, H., Erb, (Arr.), SA, Lawson-Gould/G, Schirmer, 787.

"The Angel Gabriel," Howell, J.R. Two-part treble, Boosey and Hawkes, OC2B6256.

"The Angels and the Shepherds," Kodaly, Z., Universal (Ed.), UE 10755NJ.

"The Birds," Britten, B., Unison, Boosey and Hawkes, OCTB6524.

"The Corn Song," Holst, Two-parts, E.C. Schirmer, 1898.

"The Moon of Wintertime," Mabry, G.L., SSA, Roger Dean/Lorenz Corp., 15/1336R.

"The Piglets' Christmas," Goetz, M. Unison, Boosey and Hawkes, OCTB6402.

"There is No Rose of Such Virtue," McCray, J. SSA, National Music Pub., WHC-78.

"Three Emily Dickinson Songs" ("Heart We Will Forget Him," "Going to Heaven," "The World Feels Dusty"), Hennagin, M., SA, Walton Music Corp., M-139.

"Two Catalan Carols" ("The Son of Mary," "Frozen December"), O'Neill, J., Two-parts, Alfred, 4788.

"What Sweeter Music," Butler, E., Two-part, Curtis/Kjos Pub., C8502.

"When Christ Was Born," Pfautsch, L., SA, Wynn/Music, WMP 2201.

"Wie will ich mich freuen," (My Spirit, be Joyful), Bach, SA, E.C. Schirmer, 2507.

"Wir eilen mit schwachen, doch emsigen Schritten," (We hasten with eager yet faltering footsteps), SA, E. C. Schirmer, 2506.

Appendix E

References

Alderson, R. *Complete Handbook of Voice Training.* West Nyack, NY: Parker Publishing Co., 1979.

Alperson, E.D. "The Creation of Meaning through Body Movement." In *Clinical Psychology: Issues of the Seventies,* edited by A.L. Rabin, 158–59. Lansing, Michigan: Michigan State University Press, 1974.

Aronson, A.E. *Clinical Voice Disorders.* 3rd. ed. New York: Thieme Medical Publishers, 1990.

Barresi, A.L., and D. Bless. "The Relation of Selected Aerodynamic Variables to the Perception of Tessitura Pitches in the Adolescent Changing Voice." In *Proceedings: Research Symposium on the Male Adolescent Voice,* edited by E.M. Runfola, 97–110. Buffalo, New York: State University of New York at Buffalo Press, 1984.

Brodnitz, F.S. "On the Changing Voice." *National Association of Teachers of Singing Bulletin,* 40, no. 2 (1983): 24–26.

Cooksey, J.M. "Adolescent Male Changing Voices." In *Bodymind and Voice: Foundations of Voice Education,* edited by L. Thurman and G. Welch, 329–83. The VoiceCare Network Press, Minneapolis, Minnesota, 1990.

_____. "The Development of a Contemporary, Eclectic Theory for the Training and Cultivation of the Junior High School Male Changing Voice." Part I, "Existing Theories." *The Choral Journal* 18, no. 2 (1977a): 5–14; Part II, "Scientific and Empirical Findings: Some Tentative Solutions." *The Choral Journal* 18, no. 3 (1977b): 5–16; Part III, "Developing an Integrated Approach to the Care and Training of the Junior High School Male Changing Voice." *The Choral Journal* 18, no. 4 (1977c): 5–15; Part IV, "Selecting Music for the Junior High School Male Changing Voice." *The Choral Journal* 18, no. 5 (1978): 5–18.

_____. "Do Adolescent Voices 'Break' or Do They 'Transform?'" *Voice,* The Journal of the British Voice Association 2, no. 1 (1993): 15–39.

_____. "Male Adolescent Transforming Voices: Voice Classification, Vocal Skill Development and Music Literature Selection." In *Bodymind and Voice,* edited by L. Thurman and G. Welch, 589–609. Book V, Minneapolis, Minnesota, 1997.

_____. "Vocal-Acoustical Measures of Prototypical Patterns Related to Voice Maturation in the Adolescent Male." In *Transcripts of the Thirteenth Symposium, Care of the Professional Voice, Part II: Vocal Therapeutics and Medicine,* edited by Van L. Lawrence, 469–80. New York: The Voice Foundation, 1985.

_____. "Voice Transformation in Male Adolescents." In *Bodymind and Voice,* edited by L. Thurman, G. and Welch, 495–315. Book IV, Minneapolis, Minnesota, 1997.

Cooksey, J.M., and R.L. Beckett, and R. Wiseman. "A Longitudinal Investigation of Selected Vocal, Physiological, and Acoustical Factors Associated with Voice Maturation in the Junior High School Male Adolescent." In *Proceedings: Research Symposium on the Male Adolescent Voice,* edited by E.M. Runfola, 4–60. State University of New York at Buffalo Press, Buffalo, New York, 1984.

Cooksey, J.M., and G.F. Welch. "Adolescence, Singing Development and National Curricula Design." *British Journal of Music Education,* 15, no. 1 (1998): 99–119.

Cooper, I., and K.O. Kuersteiner. *Teaching Junior High Music.* Boston: Allyn and Bacon, Inc., 1965.

Cyrier, A. *A Study of Vocal Registers and Transitional Pitches of the Adolescent Female.* Master's thesis, University of Missouri at Kansas City, 1981.

Dickson, J.H. "The Training of Conductors through the Methodology of Kinesthetics." *The Choral Journal,* March (1992): 15–20.

Fischer, K.W. and S.P. Rose. "Dynamic Development of Coordination of Components in Brain and Behavior: a Framework for Theory and Research." In *Human Behavior and the Developing Brain,* edited by G. Guilford, and K.W. Fischer, 3–66. New York: Guilford Pub., 1994.

Frank, F., and M. Sparber. "Die Premutationsstimme, die Mutationsstimme und die Postmutationsstimme in Sonagramm" (The premutation voice, mutation voice, and the postmutation voice in the sonagram). *Folia Phoniatrica,* 22 (1970): 425–33.

Frank, F., and M. Sparber. "Stimmumfange bei Kindern aus neuer Sicht" (Vocal ranges in children from a new perspective). *Folia Phoniatrica,* 22 (1970): 397–402.

Gackle, L. "The Adolescent Female Voice: Characteristics of Change and Stages of Development." *The Choral Journal* 31, no. 8 (1991): 17–25.

Gackle, L. "Female Adolescent Changing Voices: Voice Classification, Voice Skill Development, and Music Literature Selection." In *Bodymind and Voice,* edited by L. Thurman and G. Welch, 582–88. Book V, 1997.

Gackle, L. "Understanding Adolescent Female Changing Voices." In *Bodymind and Voice,* edited by L. Thurman and G. Welch, 400–16. 1992.

Gackle, L. "Understanding Voice Transformation in Female Adolescents." In *Bodymind and Voice,* edited by L. Thurman and G. Welch, 516–21. Book IV, 1997.

Groom, M. "A Descriptive Analysis of Development in Adolescent Male Voices during the Summer Time Period." In *Proceedings: Research Symposium on the Male Adolescent Voice,* edited by E.M. Runfola, 80–85. Buffalo, New York: State University of New York at Buffalo Press, 1984.

Harries, M., M. Griffin, J. Walker, and S. Hawkis. "Changes in the Male Voice during Puberty: Speaking and Singing Voice Parameters." *Logopedics Vocology,* 21, no. 2 (1996): 95–100.

Kahane, J.C. "A Morphological Study of the Human Prepubertal and Pubertal Larynx." *American Journal of Anatomy,* 151, no. 1 (1978): 11–19.

McKenzie, D. *Training the Boy's Changing Voice.* London: Bradford and Dickens, Drayton House, 1956.

Naidr, J., M. Zboril, and K. Sevcik. "Die pubertalen Veranderungen der Stimme bei Jungen im Verlauf von 5 Jahren" (Pubertal voice changes in boys over a period of 5 years). *Folia Phoniatrica,* 17 (1965): 1–18.

Ruble, D.N. "The Experience of Menarchy." *Child Development* 53: 1557–66.

Rutkowski, J. "Final Results of a Longitudinal Study Investigating the Validity of Cooksey's Theory for Training the Adolescent Male Voice." *Pennsylvania Music Educators Association Bulletin in Music Education,* 16 (1985): 3–10.

Rutkowski, J. "Two-Year Results on a Longitudinal Study Investigating the Validity of Cooksey's Theory for Training the Adolescent Male Voice." In *Proceedings: Research Symposium on the Male Adolescent Voice,* edited by E.M. Runfola, 86–97. Buffalo, New York: State University of New York at Buffalo Press, 1984.

Swanson, F. *Music Teaching in the Junior High and Middle School.* Englewood Cliffs, New Jersey: Prentice-Hall, Inc., 1973.

Thatcher, R.W. "Cyclic Cortical Reorganization: Origins of Human Cognitive Development." *Human Behavior and the Developing Brain,* edited by G. Dawson and K.W. Fischer, 232–66. New York: Guilford Pub., 1994.

Thurman, L., and C.A. Klitzke. "Voice Education and Health Care for Young Voices." *Vocal Arts Medicine: The Care and Prevention of Professional Voice Disorders.* 226–68. New York: Thieme Medical Publishers, 1994.

Williams, B., G. Larson, and D. Price. "An Investigation of Selected Female Singing and Speaking Voice Characteristics through Comparison of a Group of Pre-Menarcheal Girls to a Group of Post-Menarcheal Girls." *Journal of Singing,* 52, no. 3 (1996): 33–40.

Wolverton, V.D. "Classifying Adolescent Singing Voices." Ph.D. diss., University of Iowa, 1985. Abstract in *Dissertation Abstracts International.* 47 (1986): 708A.

NOTES